community paediatrics

to Elsie and George
who made childhood a joy

community paediatrics

a primer in child care

Elsie D. May

specialist in community medicine (child health)
Birmingham Area Health Authority (Teaching)

MTP PRESS LIMITED
International Medical Publishers

Published by
MTP Press Limited
Falcon House
Lancaster, England

First published 1980

British Library Cataloguing in Publication Data

May, Elsie D
Community paediatrics.
1. Community health services for children – Great Britain
I. Title
362.7′8′10941 RJ101

ISBN 0-85200-079-0

Photoset, printed and bound
in Great Britain by
REDWOOD BURN LIMITED
Trowbridge & Esher

contents

chapter one

who am I?

In the United Kingdom prior to 1837, the birth of a baby was recorded in the parish register when the parents presented their infant for the religious ceremony of baptism. After 1837, all births were notified to the Registrar General, and following the Public Health Act[1] of 1936 the notification of each birth was made known to the Medical Officer of Health, now the Area Medical Officer (AMO). The latter provision was re-enacted in the National Health Service (NHS) Act of 1977 which states that all babies born after the 28th week of pregnancy whether alive or dead should be notified to the AMO either 'at the time of, or within six hours after, the birth'[2].

Both father and mother are equally important in the development of each child as an individual and both parents play a necessary role in their child's understanding of the social, emotional and sexual mores of the family and the society in which their child is reared. In a National Child Development Study[3] of 16-year-olds in 1964, 95% of the cohort (11 600 children) were living with their natural mother though only 87% were living with their natural father. Where children are brought up by a stepfather, they may wish to retain their father's name and not assume the name of their stepfather however kindly and loved he may be. There will also be those children who will be only too glad to be relieved of the name of a parent who has forsaken them or treated them cruelly. Nevertheless the children's sense of identity by name is important and not easily destroyed.

At least 5% of children in 1964 needed to search for 'natural' parents. As the survey shows, these children have either lost their parents through death or been discarded by them. Some children will be adopted or brought up by relatives but of the survey cohort 1.4% had no regular mother figure and 7.3% had no regular father figure, a disturbing volume of childhood misery.

The figures for single parents are rising rapidly. In 1971, there were 500 000 single parents in the United Kingdom and in 1976 there were 750 000 single parent families affecting over one million children[4]. Society's attitude to the father left to bring up his children alone is usually sympathetic and helpful; the mother alone is not so well supported[5]. Single fathers may be supported by female relatives and have housekeepers, whereas single mothers are less likely to be supported by either of these groups[5].

Dr Winnicott's imagery[6] of the home as a place where the father creates security and space for the mother to care for their child shows the importance for both parents and children of feeling secure and the necessity of security for mothering and good child care in normal child development. Children need the security of knowing where they belong as well as the security of knowing to whom they belong. It is distressing to hear professional workers talking to children about 'home' as being the place where their parent(s) live when, to the child, 'home' is the children's home or foster home if their parents have shown little or no interest in the child.

The birth of a handicapped child is a frightening prospect for parents and their initial reaction will be grief and feelings of rejection which they must be given the opportunity to discuss. Three states or crises[7] have been described of parents' reactions to their handicapped child: the first, shock and grief; secondly, a value crisis when the parents have to refashion their hopes for the child's future; and thirdly, after months and often years a reality crisis when they come to grips with the problem. The rearing of a handicapped child will be more expensive socially, emotionally and financially for the family and this is acknowledged in the United Kingdom by special allowances. It is also more expensive for the country in which the handicapped child lives, on social, health and educational grounds.

table 1

perinatal mortality – stillbirths and deaths under 1 week per 1000 total births

Year	*England and Wales*	*Finland*	*France*
1960	33.5	25.3	31.8
1965	27.3	22.3	24.3
1970	23.5	17.2	20.7
1974	20.35	14.6	19.3

from *Demographic Yearbook, 1966, pp. 264–5*

With improved family planning and falling birthrate the prevention of handicap is of increasing importance. In France a system of allowances payable to mothers when they keep their appointments for antenatal and infant health care has been introduced and there has been a considerable fall in perinatal mortality (table 1). A similar fall has occurred in Finland and in England and Wales, where free antenatal care, hospital delivery, postnatal care and child health care are available[8].

To assess the results of the French programme, an evaluation of the epidemiology of perinatalogy[9] was undertaken in the Rhône-Alpes region between 1972 and 1975. No significant change was found in the number of mothers who attended for their first consultation early in pregnancy (i.e. in the first trimester) but significantly more mothers (from 45.8% to 53.3%) attended the antenatal clinic on more than four occasions throughout their pregnancy. There has been a notable improvement in the quality of prevention in antenatal care. The survey showed no change in the numbers of premature births, either by gestational age or birth weight, and no fall in the number of congenital anomalies. There was however a significant reduction from 23.8% to 15.6% in pathology due to complications of pregnancy and childbirth.

Perinatal deaths are all stillbirths and deaths occurring in the first week of life. If we accept the statement that perinatal death is a crude measure of near death[10], a reduction in perinatal mortality due to the complications of pregnancy and delivery (accounting for 45% of perinatal deaths in the United Kingdom[11]) should lead to a reduction in morbidity, handicap and infant death due to these causes. The French ascribe 65% of handicap to perinatal causes whereas paediatricians in the United Kingdom working with children with chronic neurological handicap do not find such frequently convincing evidence of known factors operating during the perinatal period, and where there is an abnormal presentation or difficulty in labour this is more likely to occur in the presence of congenital anomalies, the small baby or maternal toxaemia.

Infant deaths are all deaths in the first year including the late neonatal deaths, i.e. from 1 week to 4 weeks of life. The infant death rate in England and Wales has not shown the same rate of fall as other European countries (table 2) despite free health services for parents and their infants. After the first week of life, congenital anomalies play a small role in infant death – 40% of infant deaths in Birmingham (England) in 1977 were cot deaths or sudden infant death syndrome (SIDS) – and although absolute numbers are falling with the fall in the birthrate (the Birmingham birthrate[12] was 21 707 in 1965 and 13 540 in 1975) the proportion of deaths due to SIDS appears to be remaining constant. It is reported that the best chance of surviving the first year of life in the United Kingdom is to be born between March and June, the worst time being November due to respiratory infection[13]. These seasonal variations, and deaths due to respiratory disease, do not apply to Finland or Sweden. As parents now plan their families perhaps they should be warned of this marked seasonal variation.

table 2

infant mortality – deaths under one year per 1000 live births

Year	*England and Wales*	*Finland*	*France*
1960	21.8	21.0	27.4
1965	19.0	17.6	21.9
1970	18.2	13.2	18.2
1974	16.35	11.0	14.7

points on screening normal development and routine medical examination

Paediatrics is concerned with producing healthy adults and its basic science is the study of growth and development[14]. The height of children is related to their birthweight, mother's height and mother's parity[15]. Perinatal mortality is higher in short mothers than in tall mothers even in the same social class[11]. As birthweight is closely related to mother's stature and low birthweight is a major cause of perinatal mortality, environmental factors contributing to short stature should be amended if possible. It is considered that genetic endowment and social environment govern attained height and intelligence[16]. A study of children aged 5–11 years in England and Scotland[17] showed that father's unemployment and sibship size had a significant effect on the height of the children, who were shorter. Similarly, in Scotland, sibship size affected the height of children in all social groups. Social class does not appear to affect the growth and maturation of adolescents in Sweden[18].

history and examination

History taking and recording are useful so long as a routine is followed and essential information is not omitted. All records including investigations and treatment will become legally more important with legislation to protect the health and welfare and development of children both pre- and post-natally[19].

An unsolicited medical examination, whether in the clinic or the school, will cause some children to show excessive shyness and even fear, calling for special expertise and care on the part of the doctor and nurse involved. With patience, skill and explanation, most children become willing and co-operative. Rarely a child will need one or more visits to watch other children being examined (with the permission of their parents), such as one psychiatrically disturbed small boy who 'helped' at his school medicals on many occasions before he would agree to undress and allow himself to be examined. There was an equally long interval before he was weaned from undressing each time he saw the school doctor's car arrive at school.

A different situation presents itself at special schools for handicapped children. These children have often been exposed to a number of doctors, nurses and frequent hospital visits. Faced with another examination at school, superficially the child may appear confident, but this attitude may mask a feeling of harassment and insecurity. A relaxed parent coupled with an explanation given gently even to the youngest child will help to reassure them that the examination will not presage injections or admission to hospital.

Before seeing the doctor, the nurse will have recorded details of the family history, both social and medical, as well as the child's early history including details of the pregnancy and delivery and the child's health since that time as related by the parents. The child's height, weight and skull circumference are recorded on charts (figures 1–4). Routine urine testing and screening for bacteriuria is necessary only in the child under 4 years of age.

Prior to coming into the doctor's room, the child will be

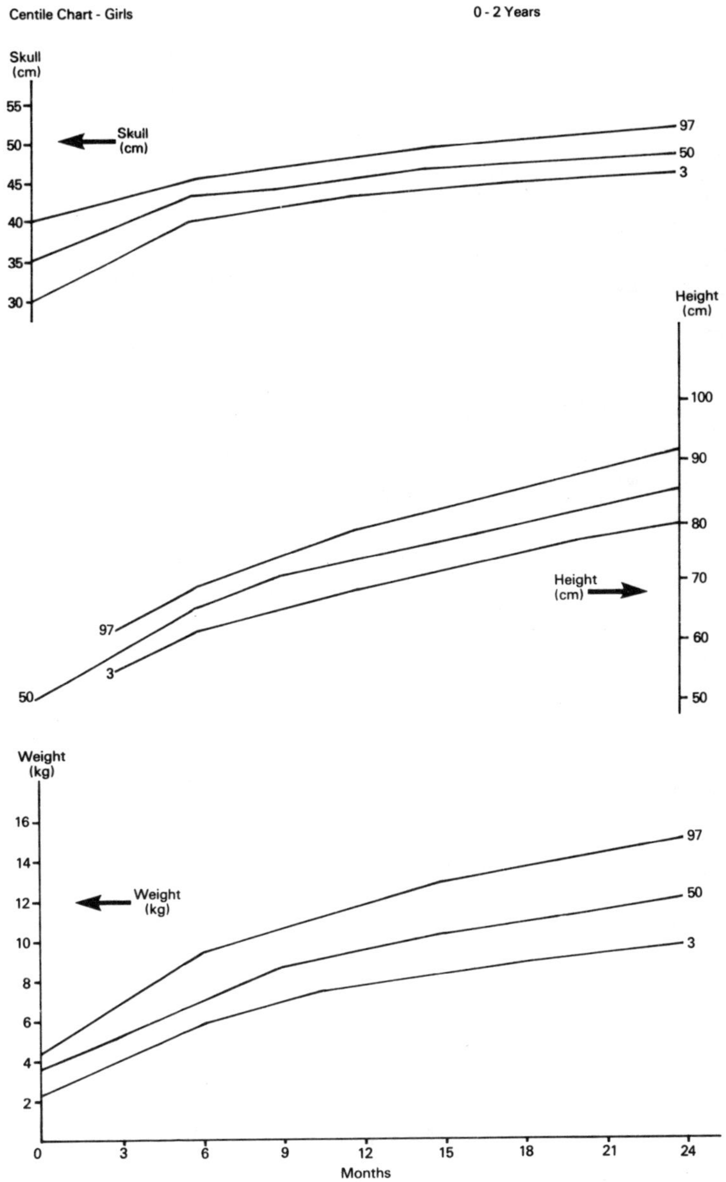

figure 1
centile chart – girls 0–2 years

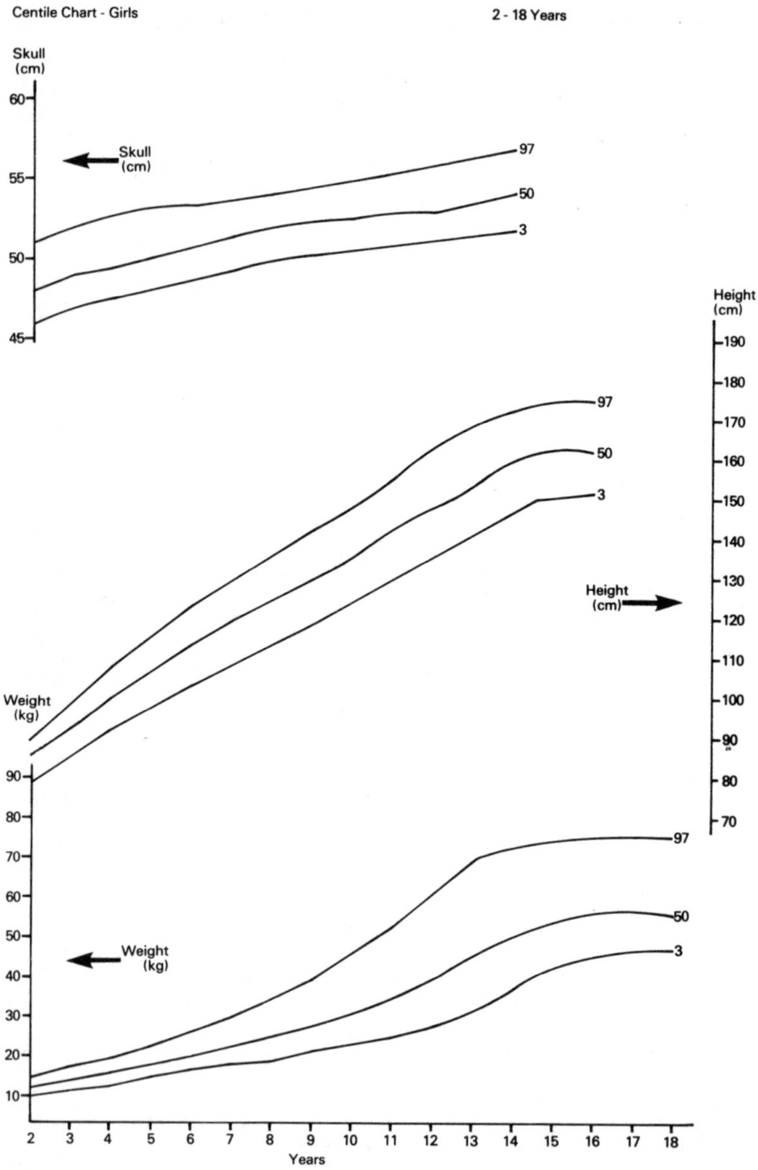

figure 2
centile chart – girls 2–18 years

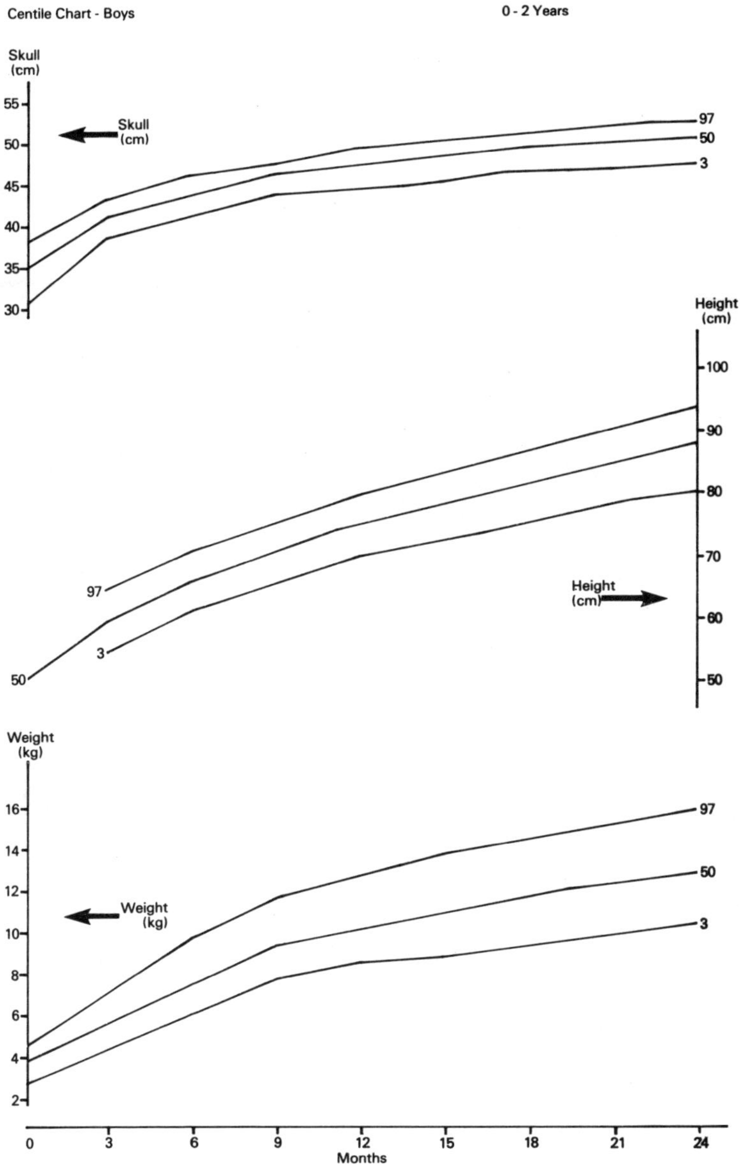

figure 3
centile chart – boys 0–2 years

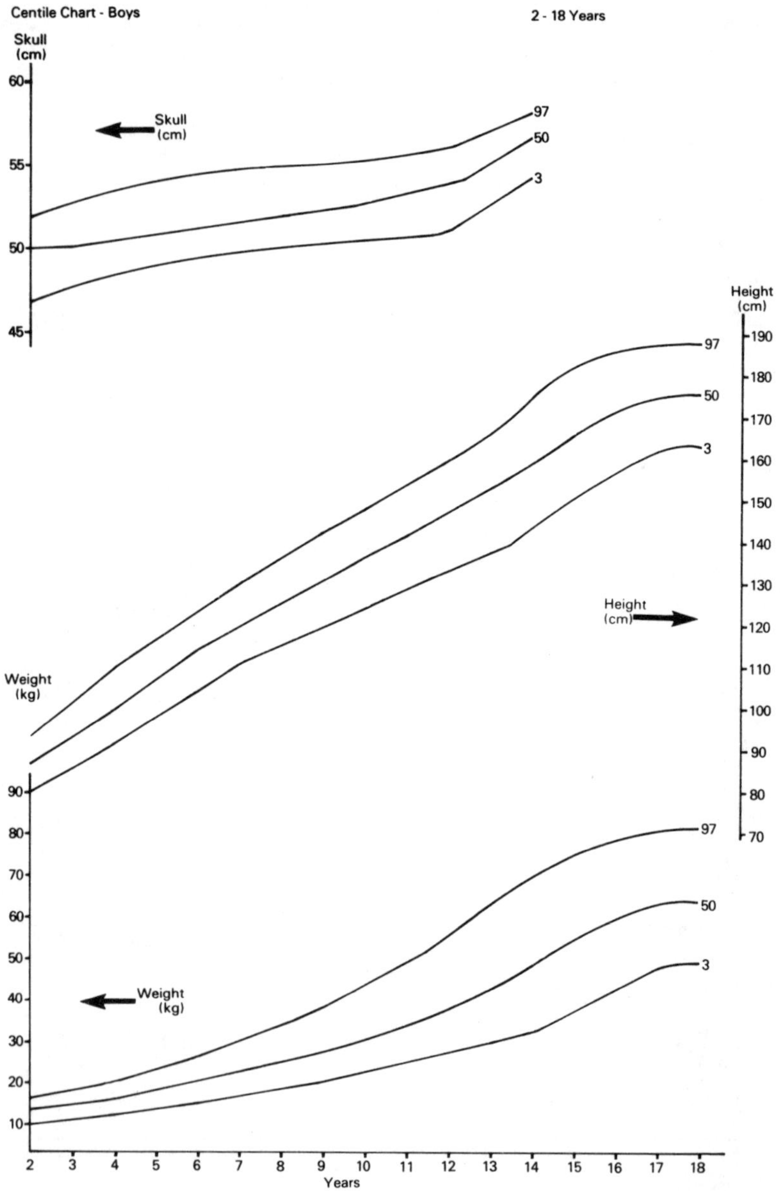

figure 4
centile chart – boys 2–18 years

undressed. It is preferable at routine examinations to leave babies and young children under the age of seven years dressed in their vests/singlets, nappies/underpants and socks. Nakedness makes some small children feel vulnerable and therefore nervous. With children under two years, by leaving the child only partly undressed, the doctor can observe the mother's handling of her child in the act of undressing and with older children the doctor can observe *how* the child manages and *whether* the child can manage these often difficult garments. Underclothing and socks deserve additional attention as they may be too small and too tight causing constriction, pain and deformity.

After greeting the mother and the child, allow the child to stay near the mother and to sit on her knee if necessary. The doctor should suggest the latter if the need arises, as some mothers are shy of behaving naturally at medical examinations. The child should be allowed to play with toys while the doctor discusses the history, elaborating on any details that appear significant or cause concern to the parents. The number of siblings and birth order should be noted, including the schools the siblings attend. Parents on occasion do conceal handicap in a sibling but quite happily divulge the name of the school the child attends and so alert the doctor who can then probe the area delicately. As well as the schools the siblings attend and the parents' attitude to those siblings where there are particular educational problems, it is often worthwhile knowing which schools the parents themselves attended as children. The procedure during the examination is then explained to the parent(s) and they are asked not to reply to questions directed by the doctor to their son or daughter unless specifically asked to do so.

The child is now relaxed and undressing can be completed. Asking the child to sit on the floor to take off his socks is a useful way of observing motor development. During this period observe the general demeanour, posture and behaviour of the child and the parent. In examining a child or an adolescent, the first approach is to examine the hands and upper limbs. This is a less threatening gesture than examination of the head and neck, whether the patient is on an examination couch or not. When the child is put on the examination couch the parent must be invited to stand by the couch. Once the examination of the upper limbs is completed, one can proceed with whichever routine is preferred. A routine is necessary as one is looking for an abnormality or anomaly of development, health and behaviour in a normal population.

The development of each infant progresses from conception to adulthood, and neurologically occurs in a cephalocaudal fashion as the higher centres in the cerebral cortex inhibit the primitive responses. Primitive responses are mass reactions which affect the whole body, as in the Moro response (p. 14), but which are variable and depend on the state of the infant, in contradistinction to a reflex such as the knee jerk which when elicited is always the same[20] (tables 3 and 4). Primitive responses can be observed in the fetus as early as 10 weeks gestation following touch stimulation, and reflex sucking has been observed at 24 weeks gestation. Inhibition of these involuntary responses by the higher centres in

table 3

			primitive responses
Grasp – hand		–	birth to 3 months
Grasp – foot		–	birth to 9 months
Rooting		–	birth to 3 months
Moro		–	birth to 3 months
Asymmetric tonic neck		–	birth to 3 months
Primary stepping		–	birth to 2 months
Foot placing		–	birth to 2nd year
			secondary responses
Balance		–	at 10 weeks
Rolling		–	at 4 months
Protective reactions	– downward parachute	–	at 4 months
	forward parachute	–	at 6 months
	propping reaction		sideways – at 7–8 months
			backwards – at 10–12 months

table 4
spinal reflexes

anal	present at birth
ankle and plantar	present at birth
withdrawal	present at birth
biceps } knee jerk }	from 2 days
cremaster	from 10 days

the brainstem and cortex occurs as early as 28 weeks gestation, and this inhibition continues throughout infancy and childhood[21].

The rate of development of each child is unique to that child, but the sequence of development is the same for every child. The rate of disappearance of the primitive responses (table 3) is a milestone in the motor development of the infant[22], and persistence of primitive responses after 6 months of age may be an important sign of delay or abnormal cerebral maturation[23]. Of the primitive responses, the Moro response never reappears once it has disappeared no matter how severe the degree of subsequent degeneration[24].

The balancing and protection responses (table 3) which succeed the primitive responses persist throughout childhood and disappear only during adolescence. At 7 to 8 years of age these responses may be seen in the involuntary extension of the wrist and fingers when the child is asked to walk on the outer borders of his feet. At 9 to 10 years, imitative movements may be seen in the inactive hand while the opposite hand is performing an action. Abnormalities of these associated movements are best observed in the Fog tests[25]. As well as motor development, the development of language and adaptive behaviour and conscious control of emotion are dependent on normal neurological development, and all of these attributes are necessary for mature mental and social development[21].

primitive responses (table 3)

Grasp reflex: In the first two months, the hands are normally closed with the thumb under the fingers. Pressure of an object on the palm or the palmar surface of the fingers causes tonic flexion which is reinforced if the object is withdrawn. Persistent fisting after 2 months is not normal, as the hands by this time are kept open in preparation for active prehension.

Foot: Pressure on the sole of the foot at the base of the toes causes flexion of the toes. Toe grasp disappears at 9 to 10 months in preparation for standing and walking.

Rooting: An object pressed against the infant's cheek will cause him to open his mouth and to turn his head so that he can respond in this way to the nipple or teat.

Moro: This response is elicited by jarring the cot or by the examiner letting the infant's head drop through from one hand to the other causing sudden extension. This procedure elicits sudden bilateral extension of the upper limbs followed by flexion. Absence in the neonatal period or persistence after the age of 6 months is evidence of cerebral dysfunction.

Foot placing: The infant held in vertical suspension is taken to the table and the dorsum of the foot allowed to touch the edge of the table, when the lower limb will be flexed and swung onto the table. This response becomes less vigorous but may persist into the second year. A normal placing response indicates that the muscle function of the lower limbs is normal.

Primary stepping: Having tested for placing, the infant with feet on the flat table surface is held leaning forward and will usually take a few steps.

Asymmetric tonic neck response (ATNR): When the infant turns his head to one side, or the infant's head is turned to one side by the examiner, the face, upper and lower limbs extend on that side and the occiput, upper and lower limbs on the opposite side flex.

secondary responses

Balance: From 10 weeks the infant will maintain his head and body posture in space. The head is lifted from supine to prone or extended when held in ventral suspension.

Rolling: In the early months the extensor response of the lower limbs is followed by a straightening, i.e. extension, of the trunk and head known as rightening, and in the early weeks, if the head is flexed on the trunk and the head is turned further than in the ATNR, the infant will turn his trunk to align it with the head. After 4 months this response changes. When the head is turned, the hips and lower limbs follow first then the shoulders. If the pelvis is turned first the head follows first and then the trunk.

Downward parachute: Under the age of 4 months infants, held vertically, will respond to sudden downward movement by a Moro response. After that age they will respond with extension and abduction of the lower limbs.

Forward parachute: In ventral suspension and moved forwards and downwards, the infant will extend and abduct the upper limbs and extend the fingers.

Propping:

Sideways – gently pushed to one side the infant will extend the limbs on the side being pushed and flex the limbs on the opposite side, and the trunk and neck move to counteract the displacing force.

Backward – the infant tilted backwards will extend and abduct the upper limbs behind the trunk with extended fingers, and the head will move into line with the trunk.

Any abnormality in responses will be associated with other signs. The one most commonly overlooked is hypotonia, the baby showing lack of movement and subsequently delay in development[26]. An early sign of hypotonia is the baby who, when held in vertical suspension, slips through the examiner's hands. Significant asymmetries are more likely to be noticed by observing the baby's posture and mobility than by examination of the musculature. Hypertonia is an important indication of neurological disease, but must not be mistaken for the vigorous resistance of the healthy infant to passive movement. Hypertonia will be present at rest in contrast to the relaxation of the normal infant.

The following is a list of the main developmental points to be looked for at various ages (see appendix 2):

6/52 Skull circumference, weight and length.
Raises head to the horizontal but cannot hold head in the horizontal: spinal reflexes (table 4).
Note any anomalies of the genitalia and ensure that the testicles are in the scrotum. Undescended testicles and other anomalies should be referred to the paediatric surgical clinic.
Fixed focal length for vision of 9–10 inches. The baby will follow a dangling ball or bright object from the side to the midline.
All babies should be smiling, even blind babies; if not smiling by 8 weeks specialist advice should be obtained.
Parents happy: If parents are not satisfied about their baby's progress and development, close follow-up or further specialist advice should be obtained.

6–8/12 Skull circumference, weight and length.
Rolls to prone, reaches forward with extended arms to be picked up.
Developing trunk control, recovers from a forward tilt.
Focal length is arms' length; the baby is interested in his feet as well as his hands.
Vocalization is a double sound: 'dada, baba'; single consonant sounds have already developed.
Persistence of hand regard is abnormal.

12/12 Skull circumference, weight and length.
Pulls to stand, recovers from backward tilt; has already developed righting from sideways tilt.
Focal length is equivalent to 6/18 Snellen.

Chewing has developed with lip control and tongue control. This is necessary to reject food and to drink from a cup.
Imitates sounds but cannot say words with meaning, understands 'no'.

1½–2 years Skull circumference, weight and height. (Anterior fontanelle closed at 18/12).
Begins to swing arms walking, able to pick up a toy from the ground and to walk backwards.
Focal length is now equivalent to 6/12 Snellen.
Can say two or three word phrases or combination of words; do not rely on reported speech. Parents may report their children as uttering a two or three word phrase which in popular usage has become a single word phrase, e.g. in Birmingham 'here you are' is run together to form one word 'herey' are' and in developmental terms must be counted as one word.
Dental health: 16 teeth – first visit to the dentist.
Persistent mouthing and casting between 12 and 18 months must be regarded as abnormal.

3 years Skull circumference, weight and height.
Can jump off a step and go upstairs unaided. Can dress and undress apart from difficult fastenings.
Focal length is equal to 6/9 Snellen.
Has a vocabulary of 1000 words and can repeat a 6-syllable sentence spoken slowly by the examiner facing the child. Can name common objects from pictures, such as cup, spoon, doll.

4½–5 years Skull circumference, weight and height.
Fully competent on stairs, buses, dressing and undressing.
Surgery for undescended testicles should be completed before school entry.
Focal length is now equivalent to 6/6 Snellen and vision should be tested by the Snellen chart if possible.
Hypermetropia is the more common refractive error in young children as congenital myopia is rare.

Test hearing to voice using the word lists prepared by the Manchester Audiology clinic which cover thirty speech sounds (see table 8, page 164) and a 5-year-old should score 92%.

Whenever a baby or child attends for a medical examination, notes should be made of his developmental progress as well as the results recorded at specific ages. Appendix 2 shows a set of developmental questionnaires for six weeks to five years.

Parameters of growth – skull circumference, height and weight – are measured regularly in a child under the age of two years and annually thereafter. More frequent measurement is necessary if abnormality or disparity is noted or there is a risk that the child is being neglected. A single measurement is never useful. Children's height should be measured as far as possible at the same time each day as stature decreases as the day progresses[27].

Screening of hearing takes place at 8/12, 3 years, 5 years, 9 years and 14 years of age. It has been suggested that infants come 'pre-wired' to make many if not all speech discriminations. To test this ability in infants a visually reinforced speech discrimination test (VRISD) was used on babies aged 3 months compared with babies aged 6 and 12 months[28]. The results suggest that listening experience is necessary to discriminate all sounds. The partially hearing baby and the baby with a unilateral hearing loss are the ones most commonly missed on present screening procedures, to their detriment. The nose and throat and tympanic membranes are reviewed at every examination in childhood.

It is not possible to test visual acuity objectively in normal children before 3–5 years of age. Both distant and near vision is assessed at every examination in the handicapped child as important clues may be missed if the handicapped child is unable to co-operate at a single examination. Schoolchildren at ordinary schools have their vision, both distant and near, tested yearly or every two years, and their colour vision tested using the Ishihara test[29] in the primary school usually at 10 years of age.

Serious congenital anomalies will be excluded by examination, including examination of the fundi. Screening tests for squint include:

(1) Examination of the corneal reflection,

(2) A cover test for squint, and

(3) Examination of ocular movements.

Corneal reflections are examined by getting the baby to look at a low-intensity bulb or torch and noting the reflections in the pupil. The baby must be looking forward with head erect and the light held in the midline.

When orthoptists screen young children for squint they will test binocular fixation, the fixation of each eye separately, the effect of a prism and the effect of covering each eye separately. Once specialist examination has been completed there is no need to repeat tests for squint.

Children under the age of 7 years should have all their screening tests in the morning as the failure rate rises in the afternoon and leads to an increase in false positives and parental anxiety. Glasses and hearing aids should always be examined for function and fit. A rudimentary knowledge of how to correct the fit and of minor repairs needed for glasses and hearing aids is a useful attribute in a children's doctor.

Heart murmurs are not uncommonly found in children at routine examination. If the murmur is thought to be pathological, the child would be referred via the family doctor for further investigation and treatment at the specialist paediatric cardiology clinic. The innocent murmur will be kept under review either by the school doctor or the family doctor if they are not the same person. It is not usual practice to tell parents when their child has an apparently innocent murmur as this tends to create unnecessary anxiety. If the murmur is still present at a follow-up examination then, in consultation with the family doctor, the parents would be told and arrangements made for the child to be seen at the paediatric cardiology clinic. If the innocent nature of the murmur is confirmed, but the murmur is present at the adolescent examination, the school doctor would let the family doctor know and suggest a further referral, in preparation for the pupil's future employment and to exclude contra-indications.

With very young children there may not be sufficient co-operation to test rapid movements but as soon as possible this should be tested with finger tapping and rotatory movement of the forearms, to see that the child is able to perform these movements efficiently. Dysdiadochokinesia is a symptom of ataxic cerebral palsy, the most commonly missed type of the disorder.

Once normal growth and development have been accomplished and there are no serious intercurrent illnesses or accidents affecting the individual child, repeated physical examination is unnecessary.

References

1. The Public Health Act (1936). (London: HMSO)
2. National Health Service Act (1977). (London: HMSO)
3. Fogelman, K. (1976). *Britain's Sixteen-year-olds.* (London: National Children's Bureau)
4. OPCS (1977). *Social Trends.* (London: HMSO)
5. Ferri, E. (1973). Characteristics of motherless families. *Br. J. Soc. Work,* **3**, 91
6. Winnicott, D. W. (1957). *The Child and the Family: First Relationships.* (London: Tavistock Publications)
7. Wolfensburger, W. (1968). In Baumeister, A.A. (ed.) *Mental Retardation: Appraisal, Rehabilitation and Education.* (London: University of London Press)
8. Wynn, M. and Wynn, A. (1974). *The Protection of Maternity and Infancy.* (London: Council for Children's Welfare)
9. Rumeau-Roquette, C., Crost-Deniel, M., Breart, G. and du Mazau-Brun, C. (1977). Evaluation épidémiologique du programme de Sante en perinatologie. *Rev. Epidemiol. Sante Publ.*, **25**, 107
10. Nixon, W. C. W. (1963). Foreword to Butler, N. R. and Bonham, D. G. (eds.), *Perinatal Mortality: First Report of the 1958 British Perinatal Mortality Survey* (Edinburgh: Livingstone)
11. Butler, N. R. and Bonham, D. G. (1963). *Perinatal Mortality: First Report of the 1958 British Perinatal Mortality Survey.* (Edinburgh: Livingstone)
12. Neale, A. B. and Haine, G. (1976–77). *Abstract of Annual Statistics: Birmingham Statistics*, No. 19. (Birmingham: Central Statistical Office).

13. Weatherall, R. (1976). Recent seasonal patterns of infant mortality in England and Wales. In OPCS, *Child Health, A Collection of Studies.* (London: HMSO)
14. Leader (1978). Nature and nurture in child growth. *Br.Med.J.*, **1**, 322
15. Goldstein, H. (1971). Factors influencing height of 7-year-old children: results from the National Child Development Study. *Hum. Biol.*, **43**, 92
16. Tanner, J. M. (1966). Galtonian eugenics and the study of growth: the relation of body size, intelligence test score and social circumstances in children and adults. *Eugen. Rev.*, **58**, 122
17. Rona, R. J. Swan, A. V. and Altman, D. G. (1978). Social factors and height of primary schoolchildren. *J. Epidemiol. Community Health*, **32**, 147
18. Lindgren, G. (1976). Height weight and menarche of Swedish urban schoolchildren with relative socio-economic and regional factors. *Ann. Hum. Biol.*, **3**, 501
19. Law Commission (1974). *Report on Injuries to Unborn Children.* (London: HMSO)
20. MacKeith, R. C. and Robson, P. (1970). Postural reactions in the first year of life. *Update*, 1275
21. Ingram, T. T. S. (1973). Concepts and practice in paediatric neurology, In Forfar, J. O. and Arneil, G. C. (eds.). *Textbook of Paediatrics* (Edinburgh: Livingstone).
22. Prechtl, H. F. and Beintema, D. (1964). *The Neurological Examination of the Full Term Newborn Infant.* (London: Heinemann)
23. Paine, R. S. and Oppe, T. E. (1964). *Neurological Examination of Children.* (London: The Spastics Society and Heinemann)
24. Paine, R. S., Brazelton, T. D., Donovan, D. E., Drorbaugh, J. E., Hubbell, J. P. and Sears, E. M. (1964). Evolution of postural reflexes in normal children and in the presence of chronic brain syndromes. *Neurology*, **14**, 1036
25. Fog, E. and Fog, M. (1963). Cerebral inhibition examined by associated movements, In Bax, M. and MacKeith, R. C. (eds.) *Minimal Cerebral Dysfunction.* (London: Spastics Society and Heinemann)
26. Dubowitz, V. (1969). *The Floppy Infant.* (London: Heinemann).
27. Strickland, A. L. and Shearin, R. B. (1972). Diurnal height variation in children. *J. Paediatr.*, **80**, 1023
28. Eilers, R. E., Wilson, W. R. and Moore, J. M. (1977). Developmental changes in speech discrimination in infants. *J. Speech Hear. Res.*, **20**, 766
29. Ishihara, S. (1971). *Tests for Colour-Blindness.* (Tokyo: Kanehara Shuppan Co. Ltd.)

chapter two

the first year

birth and the perinatal period

Maternal nutrition, placental sufficiency and length of gestation are recognized as the most important factors in the intrauterine period of fetal life for the future physical and mental development of the baby[1,2]. In many maternity units, these factors are monitored by oestriol estimation as a measure of placental function[3], and ultrasound cephalometry as a measure of fetal growth[4]. Associated factors of importance are good maternal health, maternal age between 20 and 35 years, avoidance of drugs including cigarettes and alcohol, and regular antenatal care[5].

The highest stillbirth and perinatal mortality occurs amongst babies born too early and too small. Spontaneous premature labour and delivery may cause high perinatal mortality due to prolonged or severe intrapartum asphyxia[6], as preterm delivery due to obstetric intervention is not associated with a high perinatal mortality[7]. Small babies can be divided into two categories:

(1) The baby is delivered before term and is therefore premature. Normal growth has been achieved for gestational age.

(2) The baby shows growth retardation for its gestational age and is variously described as small-for-dates (SFD) or light-for-dates (LFD). The baby's growth retardation is due to intrauterine deprivation of oxygen and calories. These babies are malnourished whether or not they appear wasted and as they lack carbohydrate reserves they suffer from hypoglycaemia[8].

To differentiate the two groups, observation of the creases on the soles of the feet is one of the most reliable characteristics. At 36 weeks there are one or two transverse creases and these increase to cover the sole of the foot by full term. The creases develop more slowly in negro infants[9]. More detailed methods of assessment of gestational age have been described[10,11].

It has been suggested that the number of very small infants born in England is declining and that the fall is not in proportion to the fall in the birthrate but is probably due to the obstetrician's skill in controlling spontaneous, premature labour[12]. However this trend is not found in Scotland and Wales. Overall the proportion of babies weighing less than 2500 g at birth has actually increased nationally in the ten-year period 1965–74[13]. A recent survey of small-for-dates infants suggests that they can develop average potential and this may be closely related to the type of feeds offered. Breast-fed infants may take up to 270 ml kg^{-1} d^{-1} catching up their centiles at about 3 months of age[14]. Bottle-fed babies, due to our fears of obesity may receive too little milk and hence suffer prolonged malnutrition.

The important 'at risk' factors during delivery are:

(1) Abnormal presentation

(2) Difficult forceps

(3) Breech delivery

(4) Very rapid or prolonged second stage of labour.

To reduce these risks for the mother and her baby, it is necessary to persuade antenatal patients to visit their doctor and midwife early in pregnancy and to attend follow-up clinics regularly. It is incumbent on the doctor and the midwife to give expert help and to show consideration and understanding of the problems their antenatal patients may be experiencing. With improved antenatal care and accurate charting of the pelvic outlet, measurement of the fetal heart in labour by intrauterine methods and early surgical intervention when necessary will help to reduce the 'at risk' factors for the baby and the mother.

In the neonatal period, expert paediatric care for the very small (i.e. less than 2500 g), apnoeic or ill baby is essential and since 1965 active and intensive care has been practised in all special care units in Britain[15]. Recognition of the early signs of disease, the importance of diagnosis and the technical skill involved in giving (and if necessary withholding) intensive care in very small or sick newborn infants must be left in the hands of a skilled paediatrician for the sake of the baby and the family involved[16]. It is an essential part of the care of the newborn for obstetricians and paediatricians involved in neonatal care to have a close working relationship.

Both the Department of Health and Social Security (DHSS)[17] and the Report of the Committee on the Child Health Services[15] recommend specialist regional centres to provide intensive care for the newborn when special care units in district general hospitals have not the staff nor the facilities to cope efficiently with intensive care. The end result for the baby and the mother might be more serious if long distances are involved in the transfer of the very sick infant to regional centres. The possibility of transferring the mother with her baby might have to be considered, or early diagnosis and transfer of the mother for delivery of her baby.

feeding

Discussion on infant feeding should be undertaken with every mother in the antenatal clinic as soon as the pregnancy has been confirmed. Regular examination of the breasts is an integral part of the antenatal examination and any problems arising from changes in the nipples and the breasts in pregnancy should be dealt with as they arise.

Breast milk is far superior to any other form of milk feed for the human baby both nutritionally and chemically[18]. Breast milk, due to the presence of lactoferrin and secretory immunoglobulin A (IgA), protects young infants from gastroenteritis, still a potent cause of death in babies under one year[19]. Breast milk, unlike cow's milk, produces an acidic stool in which *Escherichia coli* does not thrive. The lymphocytes which produce IgA in breast milk are derived from the mother's gastrointestinal tract, the most likely source of contact with infection in the very young baby, while lactoferrin in the presence of IgA combines with iron and by removing the free iron from the baby's gastrointestinal tract prevents bacteria, including *E. coli*, from multiplying.

Though containing less calcium, phosphorus and vitamin D than cow's milk, rickets is more likely to occur in the bottle-fed baby than the breast-fed baby unless the mother is suffering from low vitamin D intake[20]. Neonatal hypocalcaemia occurs almost exclusively in babies fed on cow's milk[21]. Cow's milk, but not breast milk, contains B-lactoglobulin which is the commonest cause of milk allergy, occurring in 0.3–7% of children[22]. Where mothers are breast feeding, the prescription of medicines should be strictly limited as the secretion of prescribed medicines in breast milk may harm the developing infant.

Breast-fed infants should be weighed regularly until feeding is well established to ensure an adequate intake by volume over the 24 hours. Mothers with first babies may need encouragement to feed their babies when necessary and not necessarily on a strict schedule. If possible, breast feeding should be continued for 4 to 6 months or longer if the mother and baby wish to do so. Mothers who find breast feeding difficult might manage a shorter period such as the first two weeks of the baby's life; even such a short period will create advantages for the future immunological and emotional development of the baby. No mother should be asked to persevere with breast feeding her baby if this is difficult, unsatisfactory or repugnant to her.

Cow's milk for bottle feeding is an acceptable substitute for breast milk. Following the recognition of the serious biochemical disturbance which may ensue in dehydration causing hypernatraemia when babies were fed on full cream cow's milk, new formulae were produced which substantially reduced the solute load on the infant's kidneys and contained a better chemical balance. The main changes have been reductions in sodium, phosphorus and protein content[21]. Babies fed on these new formulae have serum values for calcium, urea and urine osmolarity similar to breast-fed babies.

The main proprietary brands of low-solute milks are Cow and Gate Premium, Ostermilk Complete Formula and SMA 26. A recent trial of modified Carnation milk[23] appears to show as good or better results biochemically and in the physical development of the babies. Either lactose or sucrose may be used as added sugars[24]. If cow's milk allergy occurs, breast milk or hydrolysed milk protein formulae is used for bottle feeding as there is often an associated allergy to soya-based formulae.

Once feeding has become established, the normal infant will gain weight at a rate of 30–35 g/day decreasing to 20 g/day at 6 months and 10–15 g/day by 9 months old. A baby will double his birth weight by 5 months and treble his birth weight by 12 months of age[20].

The mentally handicapped mother often has difficulty in feeding her baby and needs either considerable professional help or the continual support of grandparents and other members of the family and often both groups of people are needed. In an emergency the baby may need to be taken into care. This situation arose following the admission of an elderly lady to hospital with a varicose ulcer, leaving her mentally handicapped daughter alone at home caring for her illegitimate baby. A visit by the health visitor found the baby underfed and being offered sausage sandwiches as a feed when he was not fully weaned. The girl's married sister who lived nearby had made valiant attempts to help without success. The baby was admitted to care until the grandmother was discharged from hospital. The girl dearly loved her baby and visited him every day while he was in care, giving the staff the opportunity to help her learn how to care for her baby. When taking a history from the mentally handicapped mother to discover how she is feeding her baby, one must make detailed enquiry about the type and quantity of food being offered.

If a baby is slow to suck and feed, any mother will feel inadequate and the baby will be at risk of battering. With the mentally handicapped mother there is a dual risk – of battering, because the mother is less able to express herself and talk about her difficulties, and of infection, due to the mother's impatience with sterilization procedures and a tendency to keep the milk overlong in the baby's bottle. An extreme example of the latter was a mother's habit of keeping her baby's bottle warm between feeds by sitting the baby on it.

Vitamins A, C and D and iron are added to all commercially produced milks used in infant feeding[21]. Iron is necessary for all premature babies whether breast- or bottle-fed. Additional vitamins should be given to all babies from six weeks until five years of age. The most convenient form of giving vitamin supplements, and the one in general use, is as vitamin drops which are provided in infant health clinics or on prescription from the family doctor. Reliance on bought fruit juices and sweet blackcurrant drinks for vitamin C intake should be avoided as they encourage a liking for sweet foods, and, when used as comforters over prolonged periods, as in short drinks, may lead to dental caries. The recommended daily dose of vitamins is vitamin A 300 mg as retinol, vitamin C 30 mg and vitamin D 10 mg as cholecalciferol[18].

If, as citizens, we are serious about encouraging breast feeding, both in developed and underdeveloped countries, we must insist that governments make breast feeding financially feasible for mothers who have to work whether they are married or single. Kwashiorkor has begun to appear in the early months of infancy in Jamaica and South Africa when mothers are forced to wean their babies early in order to return to work. In 1974, 6 babies died of malnutrition and 6 died of avitaminosis in Cape Town in the first year of life[25].

If, as doctors, we are serious about encouraging breast feeding, then early contact, preferably immediately after delivery, should be established between mother and baby with the baby unclothed so that the mother and child can explore each other. Later, the mother and her baby should be nursed together, allowing early contact with the father also. Early suckling will help to stimulate breast feeding and closer attachment between mother and child: this closer attachment is still noticeable after two years[26].

A better visual presentation of breast feeding, equal in attractiveness to the posters produced for the commercial baby milks, should be displayed in all antenatal clinics and cubicles to ease the embarrassment many mothers and fathers feel in thinking and talking about breast feeding.

weaning

Weaning can be difficult and is an important time in the emotional development of the baby and in the baby's relationship with the mother, so additional support by the health visitor or the doctor may be needed until the new regime is established.

A baby will grow and develop normally if fed on milk alone with added iron and vitamins up to 4–6 months and it is recommended that the introduction of solid foods should be delayed until then[18]. Undoubtedly some babies will be hungry before this time and solids may be added to their diet. Small amounts of cereal or rice, added to the bottle feed or by spoon, are first introduced with a gradually increasing variety of food. From 2–3 months, all babies can be introduced to various tastes at family meal times, such as egg yolk, potato and gravy and apple puree, care being taken not to add extra salt, and avoiding gluten-containing foods until the baby is 6 months of age.

Asian mothers in the United Kingdom tend to regard tinned baby food, which is expensive, as superior to their own dishes and need continual reassurance that it is better to feed their babies with suitably prepared food which is cooked for the other members of their family. Where the family are vegetarian, this penchant for tinned foods may be dangerous for the baby, as the mothers tend to buy and feed their babies on cans of puddings in order to avoid meat and meat products. Excellent books, describing Asian foods and their use in infant feeding, are available in the United Kingdom and are issued to all health staff. The high incidence of rickets in the Asian community may be due to poor feeding as much as to inadequate intake of vitamin D.

During weaning, bottled cow's milk from a cup can be substituted for a bottle or breast feed until the baby is fully weaned on to cow's milk and three meals a day. Mothers should be advised not to add extra sugar or salt to any of their baby's food, as this increases the solute load on the infant kidney and may predispose the baby to obesity, and, in adult life, to hypertension. Regular measurement of growth compared with centile charts (figures 1–4) should be used to monitor a baby's diet and advise the mother on feeds.

Extra drinks of water (which must be boiled for young babies and for everyone where water supplies are doubtful) should be given between feeds if the baby is thirsty in very hot weather or if infection is present.

screening

Shortly after birth, every newborn infant is subjected to a short period of intensive observation and examination to confirm his or her normality. Two important screening tests are carried out within the first ten days after birth – the first to exclude congenital dislocation of the hip; the second to exclude phenylketonuria (PKU), an inherited metabolic disorder.

screening for congenital dislocation of the hip

The occurrence of congenital dislocation of the hip is from 3–6 per 1000 live births[27]. The introduction of routine screening in the neonatal period by Von Rosen[28], Barlow[29], and Coleman[30] was intended to prevent the occurrence of late recognition, with the possibility of serious deformity, when a child starts to walk. However the latter may, in some cases, be due to late dislocation. Clinical examination, using the method of Ortolani[31] or Barlow[29], is carried out with the baby warm, fed and relaxed, lying on his back on a firm surface. The hips are flexed to a right angle and the knees fully flexed into the palm of the examiner's hand. The middle finger of each hand is placed over the greater trochanter and the thumb is applied to the inner side of the thigh opposite the lesser trochanter (figure 5). The thighs are abducted using a gentle movement while the middle finger presses the greater trochanter forward – if the hip is dislocated the femoral head can be felt and heard to slip into the acetabulum in the mid-range of abduction.

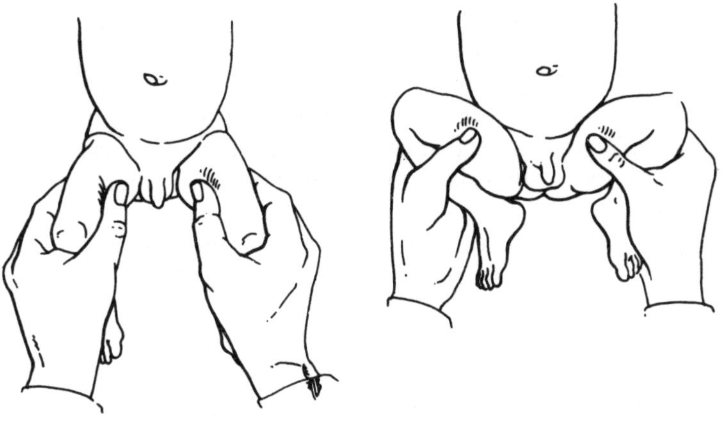

figure 5
examination for congenital dislocation of the hip (from *Textbook of Paediatrics*, edited by J. O. Forfar and G. C. Arneil, 2nd Edn., by kind permission of the publishers Churchill Livingstone, Edinburgh)

The second stage applies gentle pressure backwards and outwards with the thumb on the inner side of the thigh. If the femoral head slips over the posterior lip of the acetabulum but returns when pressure is relased and the hip abducted, the hip is regarded as unstable but not dislocated. The diagnosis rests on careful clinical examination – X-rays are not helpful in doubtful cases[32].

It is possible to have a dislocated hip that does not reduce on abduction and where there is no jerk or thud but where abduction is restricted on one or, more often, both sides, as the condition is often bilateral[32]. Treatment of a dislocated hip requires management by an orthopaedic surgeon and generally means splinting in abduction for 2–3 months.

biochemical screening

All infants born in Britain, Eire, Europe, North America, Australia and New Zealand are screened for phenylketonuria, an inherited metabolic disorder which can be treated successfully by giving the affected baby a low phenylalanine diet as early as possible, preferably before the baby is six weeks old, and continued throughout childhood. The incidence in Caucasians is 1 in 10 000 births[33], although 1 in 5000 in Ireland and Western Scotland[34]. It is believed to be uncommon in other ethnic groups. The cause of the disorder is an inherited deficiency of liver phenylalanine hydroxylase activity, resulting in an accumulation of phenylalanine and its metabolic products. The accumulation of phenylalanine affects mental development often resulting in severe handicap which may be associated with epilepsy, behaviour disorder and eczema[35].

The test consists of collecting blood from the baby by a heel prick between the 6th and 14th days of life; earlier collection, before the 6th day, will result in false negatives as has been found in USA and Eire. The blood is collected on filter paper for a Guthrie test[36] or in a heparinized capillary tube for a Scriver test[37], and then sent to a central laboratory for testing. If the screening test is positive for phenylketonuria, the family doctor is notified and the baby admitted to hospital immediately for further investigation of blood levels and confirmation of the diagnosis, as well as the establishment of a low phenylalanine diet. The latter requires the help of an experienced dietician. Continuing advice and support for the parents is necessary from a skilled team of staff – paediatrician, clinical chemist and dietician with the support of the family doctor and health visitor.

Screening for any disease where the health services are imposing a service upon, or taking a service to, the patient, who is apparently healthy, may cause serious anxiety in the recipient[38]. This anxiety is most marked in those patients who need to be followed up but who do not need treatment. The patient found to be normal and the patient needing treatment are relieved and in favour of screening tests. The intermediate group, thrown up by all population screening methods, need to feel confident of the support and advice, not only from specialist hospital staff, but also from their family doctor and the community health staff. Time for discussion and explanation, both oral and written, is essential if patients are not to become angry and distressed especially when they are parents making decisions for their infants and children.

developmental screening

Regular developmental screening of all young children is a valuable service to the child and the parents[39]. Apart from the obvious congenital abnormalities present and recognized at birth, e.g. hare lip, cleft palate, Down's syndrome, spina bifida and hydrocephalus, regular screening is the only way to institute early therapy for other serious, crippling handicaps, e.g. cerebral palsy, hearing and vision impairment. The need to institute early therapy and the beneficial effect on the child and parents is undoubted, whereas delay often means extreme social, environmental, and even emotional deprivation, as parents are frightened to enquire about their child's delayed development in case it is due to serious mental handicap. Apparent mental retardation will be present in the educational sense if a handicapped child is deprived of appropriate play and therapy. However, given therapy, whether physiotherapy, speech therapy or specialist teaching in infancy and early childhood, a more satisfying social and emotional relationship will develop between the family and the handicapped child as well as improved developmental progress. If a handicap is not discovered in infancy, some of the deprivation can be alleviated with intensive help and specialized education once the child is admitted to school, but it is doubtful whether there is ever complete recovery. Experimental evidence shows that deprivation has serious and lasting effects on the normal child also[40].

Developmental screening, using a similar form to the charts illustrated (appendix 2) plus skull circumference, height and weight charts (figures 1–4), facilitates the recognition of two conditions which are often missed – the pretty, severely subnormal baby often presenting as a feeding problem rather than developmental delay, and the very small child presenting as a behaviour problem. Small stature, whether due to true dwarfism (unusual), emotional deprivation (more common, especially in large conurbations both in developed and undeveloped countries[41]), or mental retardation, may make a child appear very much younger than his/her chronological age, e.g. a 4-year-old may look like a 2-year-old; and the small, pretty baby may look 5–6/12 when he is in fact 10–12/12. These are ready pitfalls for the unwary. Parents will not alert the doctor either for the reasons given above or, if this is their first baby, because they are unaware of the true problem, although they will feel very bitter towards the doctor who has appeared to fail them when they become aware of the truth.

As with any tool in medicine, whether biochemical, physical or therapeutic, it is important to feel comfortable in using and assessing the results of any screening procedure. This aphorism is especially applicable to developmental screening and there is a variety of screening procedures commonly in use[42–44] as well as the one illustrated.

Many screening procedures of development can be effectively carried out by health visitors, nurses and nurses' assistants as long as they are trained to do so.

normal development

Within the first few days of life, babies can recognize their mothers by their smell[45]. At the breast, the infant and the mother share an intense experience. Whether a baby is breast- or bottle-fed, feeding offers to the baby anticipation and activity with gratification and relief of tension. Experience of excretory movements may also be accompanied by feelings of excitement and climax[46].

During the first few weeks of life, babies will cry in inverse ratio to the nursing contact they receive from their mothers. Some crying is necessary to stimulate respiratory and vocal functions[47]. Crying may be due to hunger, anger or pain. All three types of cry have a rhythmic component which is recognizable to mothers[48]. Neurologically abnormal babies have an abnormal cry, are slower to respond to a stimulus and sustain their cry for a shorter period making mothering and mutual adaptation more difficult. Cold will produce crying from the first week of life as the infant cannot shiver to retain heat[49].

When first attempting to look at an object, a baby may use first one eye and then the other, but by 3 months he will look with both eyes together. The appreciation of the separate images from each eye as a single image is binocular vision. The development of normal vision is dependent on the use and the normal function of each retina, especially the fovea, and the fusion of the images in the visual cortex (bifoveal fixation)[50]. The fovea, which contains cones only, provides distinct central vision and colour vision. The rest of the retina contains rods and cones which provide peripheral vision especially at low light intensities. Normal vision is also dependent on various mechanisms controlling motor movement. Ocular muscles· are never at rest and constantly undergo minute oscillatory movements around a central fixation point. Failure to attain normal optic fixation in the first five months of life accentuates these movements and causes life-long pendular nystagmus associated with poor visual acuity[50]. Opticokinetic nystagmus may also be present in congenital nystagmus, vividly described by one small boy when learning to read as 'catching the words as they flashed past'. Additional motor mechanisms affecting vision involve postural and proprioceptive stimuli from the muscles of the head and neck and the semicircular canals.

6 weeks: A normal baby feels comfortable in his mother's arms and will watch her face during feeding as this is the appropriate distance for social interaction for the baby's focal length. The infant learns to distinguish bright or patterned objects especially if they are moving and stand out in space and, by 2 months of age, will show greater interest in three-dimensional objects[51]. As the baby learns to know his mother as a whole human being and learns to give in return, the baby becomes a whole human being too, and the experience will be richer for the baby and the mother where the baby is breast-fed[46]. The baby will be learning to recognize his mother but will not recognize her absence[52]. There is no recognition of permanent objects because the baby is not yet able to recall them[53].

6–8 months: Although up to this age babies show evidence of distress at separation, after 6 months the distress is directed at the parents, especially the mother, and made worse by the attention of strangers[54]. The age range of onset of this social differentiation has been found to vary from 22 weeks to 15 months, with a somewhat younger onset, at about 15 weeks, in African babies[55]. There does not appear to be any correlation between onset and the nature and intensity of maternal care[54]. Fear of strangers appears between 6 and 9 months of age but is less likely to occur if the adult does not attempt physical contact and allows the infant time to assimilate a stranger[53].

The baby will now fix on an object, reach out and grasp it using the whole hand and so, by visual and tactile experience, the baby is learning to handle and mouth objects. Babies can recognize abstract objects before 6 months of age and remember shapes such as triangles, thus storing in memory the discreteness and orientation of objects prior to the acquisition of expressive speech[53].

Babbling should be established, and, although still reflex at this age, the kinaesthetic pleasure a baby receives from lip-

and tongue-movements is intensified by hearing and listening[47], a pleasure denied the deaf baby who will tend to become silent. As with vision, the use of normal neurological pathways and connections for speech and language is very important in infancy and childhood. The diagnosis of deafness, including unilateral and partial deafness, is so important and often so difficult that early involvement of the consultant otologist and the teacher of the deaf is essential when any doubt or delay exists.

Parents need to be encouraged to attend for the special tests of hearing and vision provided for their babies. The special tests of hearing made by health visitors and of vision by orthoptists are available at the infant health clinics or the family doctor's surgery. Screening for squint by orthoptists is recommended for all infants as the most effective means of preventing amblyopia, whether due to squint or unequal refractive errors (straight-eye amblyopia)[56].

12 months: Normal infants at 12 months are inquisitive and happy to explore even in unfamiliar surroundings as long as their mothers are present and easily seen. If their mothers leave them, even if another person is present, the babies' exploratory behaviour ceases, an important point in training nursery staff and child minders – acquaintance with the baby, however brief, is essential[53].

The baby is now beginning to realize that objects have an identity and a permanent existence and will look for objects when hidden[57]. As he develops speech and language, the baby learns to make sounds simulating the name of a person or an object he wants. When he utters the sound, either the person comes or the object is given to him – the first steps are taken physically and metaphorically in widening the horizon.

Simple washable toys are an important adjunct to the baby's emotional and social development. Immigrant parents, especially those who have moved from rural areas to large conurbations, need help in remembering to provide toys as play material. Alternatives to toys were easily available in their villages, and parents from rural areas forget these needs of their children in their multi-occupied, dense living conditions in large cities. Toys need to provide a range of texture and response for the baby, from the soft cuddly to the hard brick, and to be unbreakable and non-poisonous, that is chewable.

preventive medicine

immunization

The importance of immunization in preventing serious infectious disease in young children is accepted. The most difficult problem is to encourage parents to accept immunization, a series of injections, for their children and keep up the level of immunity in the community when the parents themselves have not experienced the mortality and morbidity associated with the diseases we hope to prevent. The incidence of diphtheria, tetanus and poliomyelitis is almost zero in Europe, whereas whooping cough and tuberculosis have been slower to decline. As recently as 1972, 68 000 people died of tuberculosis in Europe[58]. In the developing countries one of the greatest public health problems, due to its high incidence and mortality, is tetanus. A recent report from Iran[59] showed 150 deaths in 233 cases of neonatal tetanus. Increasing movement of populations between nations and between continents carries an increased risk of communicable disease and higher levels of immunization are important in the protection of host communities.

primary immunization

tuberculosis

BCG (*Bacillus Calmette-Guerin*) vaccine is an attenuated living strain of *Mycobacterium tuberculosis* which has been freeze dried. After reconstitution, 0.1 ml is given intradermally in the region of the insertion of the deltoid muscle.

Tuberculosis has been declining in most European countries over the last 30 years[60] due to better living conditions and BCG vaccination. Tuberculous infection in children in Europe has been diminishing at the rate of 10% per year and with the gradual disappearance of the problem, routine vaccination at any age may need to be reconsidered[60]. Immigrants and their children still form high-risk groups in many European countries. In Britain, BCG is offered to all Asian babies early in the neonatal period as the Asian population in large cities in Britain is particularly susceptible to the disease[60]. In France, tuberculosis occurs 3–5 times more frequently amongst immigrants than amongst the indigenous population[58]. BCG probably raises the level of immunity for those people who live in overcrowded conditions but may create problems, by giving a false sense of security to the physician, in the diagnosis of non-respiratory forms of tuberculosis which occur most frequently in the immigrant population[61] as the vaccine fails to protect 20% of those vaccinated.

diphtheria, pertussis, tetanus and poliomyelitis immunization

Diphtheria, pertussis and tetanus (DPT) may be given as a single injection of triple or trivalent vaccine, with oral poliomyelitis vaccine (OPV) in syrup, or, with older children and adults, on a lump of sugar. This is the primary or basic course of vaccination for all infants. Diphtheria and tetanus are given as toxoids absorbed with aluminium hydroxide which acts as an adjuvant to improve the antibody response. Pertussis is a vaccine containing killed organisms of *Bordetella pertussis*. The intramuscular route is recommended for the injection as superficial injection causes a small nodule or granuloma. Local reactions may cause a sore, red arm especially in adults and older children. Where there are contra-indications to the administration of pertussis vaccine[62] (table 5) or parents are unwilling to allow their children to receive the triple vaccine, a combined vaccine of diphtheria and tetanus is used.

The recommended interval between administration of the vaccines in the primary course of immunization is 4 to 6 weeks between the first and second dose, and 4 to 6 months between the second and third. The recommended age for starting primary immunization is 3 months and this is the practice in most countries[58]. Starting immunization at 3

table 5
contra-indications to pertussis vaccine

1	History of seizures or cerebral irritation in the neonatal period.
2	History or family history, including siblings, of epilepsy, febrile convulsions, or other disease of the nervous system.
3	Developmental or other defects.
4	Any febrile illness, particularly respiratory, until the patient has recovered.
5	Any local or general reaction to a preceding dose.

months of age will help to ensure some protection for the young infant, but for infants under 3 months of age, protection is largely dependent on older brothers and sisters being immunized. Although the antibody response to immunization is not as good at 3 months of age as it is at 6 months of age[62], there is a smaller risk of febrile convulsions as these occur most commonly between 6/12 and 3 years old[62]. In the Oxford survey[63], the rate of febrile convulsions from triple antigen was 0.09/1000 doses, whereas the occurrence of convulsions with a clinical attack of pertussis was 2/1000 children under 5 years of age. West Germany is the only developed country which does not advise routine immunization against pertussis for all children, although it is still advised for those children at risk – those living in institutions, children of large families or children with chronic lung and heart disease. Pertussis most seriously affects the very young infant[62].

Stringent attention should be paid to the contra-indications listed in the advice given by the Joint Committee on Immunisation and Vaccination[62] (table 5). Allergy, either personal or a positive family history, is no longer considered a contra-indication.

poliomyelitis

Sabin-type live virus vaccine as a means of immunization against poliomyelitis was introduced in Britain in 1962. Live virus vaccine, containing poliovirus types 1, 2 and 3, was regarded as a more acceptable means of immunization than the Salk killed vaccine which had completed successful trials earlier.

Killed vaccine has continued to be the accepted vaccine for immunization against poliomyelitis in The Netherlands, Sweden and Finland[64]. In other developed countries live vaccine remains the means of choice for the following reasons. Killed vaccine has to be given by injection whereas live vaccine is given by mouth. Killed vaccine failed to stop the spread of wild virulent viruses causing outbreaks in the United States of America[65], and a wild virulent virus may be the cause of the recent outbreak of paralytic poliomyelitis in the unvaccinated population of The Netherlands. Repeated injections of killed virus are necessary throughout childhood to maintain detectable levels of antibody to the polioviruses. Live virus, as well as being administered by mouth, multiplies in the gastro-intestinal tract inducing secretory IgA antibody and providing resistance to re-infection. This may be accompanied by a febrile illness. Live virus is antigenically potent, a single dose producing a rapid immunogenic effect, and is therefore effective in aborting epidemics[65]. There is spread by excretion and, although this form of spread carries some danger for the unvaccinated population, for the same reason it helps to maintain immunity.

Killed vaccine must be used when immunization against poliomyelitis is indicated and live vaccines are contra-indicated as in pregnancy, in patients with immunological deficiency, on steroid or immunosuppressive therapy or radiotherapy, and when patients are affected by tumours especially of the reticulo-endothelial system. Live vaccine-derived strains may be developing virulence although these are less likely to cause neurological disease[66]. Some cases of poliomyelitis have been ascribed to live vaccine; these cases are reported from the USA with a few from Europe[58]. As with triple vaccine, the level of immunization against poliomyelitis is waning in many areas, and, if children and young adults are found to have a level of immunity similar to the pre-vaccination era, there may be further serious outbreaks of the disease[66].

A survey of lameness in Ghana[67] showed an estimated incidence of poliomyelitis of 28 per 100 000, a rate comparable to that pertaining in the USA and Europe during epidemic years. In the USA, an epidemic of poliomyelitis is defined[65] as 'two or more cases caused by the same polio virus occurring in a four week period in a circumscribed population such as a city, county or metropolitan area'. High priority should be given to immunization against poliomyelitis in developing countries. The main problems in the underdeveloped countries, especially in tropical climates, are the difficulties of safety and storage for vaccines when refrigeration may be limited and, if available, may not be used effectively[68]. If killed polio vaccine is used, there are the problems of giving injections in unhygienic conditions and maintaining sterility and cleanliness. Where attempts have been made to establish immunity with live virus in African babies, this has not always been successful due, it is thought, to the high intestinal infestation rate inhibiting virus multiplication.

Rigid timing of immunization is not as important in the underdeveloped countries as the early introduction of vaccines after the baby is born. Triple antigen given to babies at birth or at one month of age showed that whooping cough was equally severe in the two groups, but more babies immunized at one month got the disease. It has also been found that the agglutinin response is the same with two widely-spaced doses (0.5 ml) of triple antigen as with three doses of antigen given at monthly intervals[68].

mortality and morbidity

The greatest modern scourges to apparently healthy babies in the first year of life are gastro-enteritis, respiratory infection, non-accidental injury (battered babies) and cot deaths (sudden infant death syndrome). In 1972, 14 000 infants between one month and one year of age were treated in hospital in England and Wales for gastro-enteritis and 410 died[69]. Respiratory infection in childhood constitutes 25% of hospital paediatrics and 55% of general practitioner consultations[70]. Of the 778 deaths[71] of children under 5 years due to acute bronchitis and bronchiolitis, over 80% occurred in the first year of life.

non-accidental injury (NAI)

Awareness of violence to young children was first noted by Caffey in 1946 when he described the association of fractures of long bones with subdural haematoma in children[72]. When it was recognized that this violence was inflicted by parents, the term 'battered child syndrome' was coined[73,74]. Boys and girls are equally affected.

Children under the age of 3 years are at greatest risk of battering and especially those under the age of 6 months where the baby is of low birth weight. There is a higher incidence of congenital abnormalities among affected children[75].

The incidence of non-accidental injury to children in the USA is thought to be 6 per thousand live births, and the 5000 cases reported each year in the United Kingdom is probably an underestimate. Of these children, 5–10% die while many more survive with permanent physical and mental handicaps, estimated at 400 new cases every year[76]. All social classes, religions and ethnic groups are responsible for inflicting pain and disability on their children in this way. The iceberg of mental cruelty can only be guessed at.

It is suggested that any injury in a child under 2 years other than a road traffic accident must always be considered a possible case of battering[77]. Where there is proven battering of a child, the finding of physical neglect in the presenting child and in the other children in the family is common, as is sibling death[78]. Although bruises and fractures are generally recognized, intraocular haemorrhage and burns are often not recognized as battering, although these are commonly found in older children[77]. Eye injuries found most commonly in battered children are periorbital bruising, with or without conjunctival and subconjunctival haemorrhage. These may occur when a blow causes a fracture of the anterior cranial fossa. There may also be anterior segment injuries, hyphaema, intraocular haemorrhage and retinal detachment. Subluxation of the lens may occur with the latter two lesions[79,80].

The following points should be looked for when there is suspicion of non-accidental injury:

(1) A succession of injuries such as bruises from pinching, bites and burns.

(2) Unexplained failure to thrive, vomiting, pyrexia and coma.

(3) All fractures in children under 2 years of age. Retinal examination and skeletal X-ray are important diagnostic aids.

(4) Serious injury to brain, retina, bones and abdominal organs which can occur without external bruising.

Parents who injure their children may show, and genuinely feel, great distress at the child's injuries but are less likely to ask how long the child will be in hospital and whether follow-up is needed or to attend follow-up appointments. The parents must be treated sympathetically but firmly in their distress. They may be evasive or contradictory in giving the history, show anger or be critical of the child for being injured, and may handle the child roughly.

Observation of the child's reactions may be helpful:

(1) Fearfulness of some adults. The child may vomit or urinate when the father's or the cohabitee's voice is heard.

(2) Miserable and clinging to the parents even when the child has been abused and rejected by them.

(3) The child may not look to his parents for comfort or want to be taken home.

(4) Apprehension when an adult approaches another crying child.

(5) Reversed caring occurs in older children with anxious watching of their mother, patting her, offering her a cigarette.

(6) Impaired ability for enjoyment with low self-esteem and behavioural adjustment symptoms. Over 50% of injured children had poor self-concepts and were *sorrowful*, unpopular children. They showed withdrawal, pseudo-adult behaviour and school learning problems.

In suspicious circumstances, where parents refuse admission to the home and to the child, there should be recourse to the local police for help without delay.

When there is overt injury, the child must be admitted to hospital immediately both for treatment and to exclude other injury. When there is suspicion of battering, a child must be seen by a doctor, preferably one who is experienced in paediatrics as it is necessary to exclude accidental injury such as that sustained at play. If there is any doubt about the severity of the injury the child should be admitted to hospital. A hospital ward is not a place of safety for a child as it is too easy to remove a child from a ward if parents are sufficiently determined and the staff are busy with other patients or visitors. As far as possible every member of staff on the ward, medical, nursing and ancillary, should be told if there is a child present who is at risk of NAI. Some Health and Social Services Departments maintain a central register of overt and suspected cases. These registers are accessible 24 hours a day to professional staff and are especially helpful to doctors in Accident and Emergency Departments when faced with a child who has a serious or suspicious injury.

In the United Kingdom, the Social Services Department must be informed in all cases of overt or suspected battering and a case conference of all the professionals involved will be held to decide what action needs to be taken to protect the child. If supervision of the family is required, that is regular visiting, this is usually carried out by a social worker but may be the health visitor/school nurse, or, where other bodies are involved, such as the National Society for the Prevention of Cruelty to Children (NSPCC) or the Probation Service, one of their officers. If it is thought necessary to remove the child to a place of safety such as a local authority children's home, evidence must be given to the magistrates, although this can be done urgently. For this reason, medical photography of any injuries that may be present, including evidence provided by the dental department on bite marks, may be of inestimable value. Forensic dentistry requires early referral to be of any value.

Stress is placed on the responsibility of social workers in dealing with the longterm follow-up of children suspected and/or recognized as battered, both as government policy and magistrates' orders. Most social work departments would admit that they have insufficient staff to adequately supervise these children and their parents, and, as the relationship between theory and practice in social work in altering parental child care practices while the child remains at home are at best unreliable[81], our expectations are unfair to the social workers and the parents involved and may be disastrous for the children.

More responsibility for the follow-up of these children should be accepted by doctors and nurses. Surveillance of children presenting with recurrent illness, failure to thrive, and in the schoolchild poor educational attainment due to recurrent illness, is more properly the province of doctors and nurses than the social worker. Ready access to consultant paediatric opinion is available in the United Kingdom.

An alternative method of supervision for the 'at risk' child, involving day care (see page 81) and giving the parents an integral role to play at the day care centre, may be more successful in those cases of suspected injury or neglect secondary to poverty and bad, overcrowded housing. To openly acknowledge that parents can feel a burst of unreasoning violence towards their children, whether they are faced with a screaming, colicky baby or an older child who appears to be deliberately stimulating anger, is a great relief to the parents concerned. It is the violence of the emotion which so shocks the parent who experiences it.

cot deaths

Cot deaths are all sudden deaths in infants reported to the coroner and may be due to any cause other than congenital anomalies. 90% of cot deaths occur after the age of one month. Several studies[82,83], have been carried out to identify specific 'at risk' factors at birth, the high-risk group being 15% of all births. The 'at risk' factors appear to be different for every community, e.g. in Britain, the Sheffield survey findings do not apply to other large cities[84], and a multicentre study is now in progress. The only common factors found in all areas are mothers aged less than 20 years with a low birth-weight baby[85]. There may well be an overlap between battering and cot death, as it was noted in the Birmingham study that four deceased siblings of battered babies had died in 'suspicious' circumstances[10]. An additional factor may be unemployment leading to poverty, increased stress on young parents and lack of attention to the baby for long periods, e.g. late rising in the morning.

The aetiological factors outlined by Valdes-Dapena[86] are suffocation, infection, hypogammaglobulinaemia, inborn errors of protein metabolism, abnormal calcium metabolism, status thymolymphaticus, adrenal or parathyroid insufficiency or hypersensitivity to cow's milk. An additional factor was postulated by Swift and Emery[87] reporting that apnoea occurred in 5–10% of sleeping newborn babies due to delay in initiation of mouth breathing after nasal occlusion during rapid eye movement (REM) sleep. The proportion of babies so affected increased at 5–7 weeks of age. Prolonged delay in initiating mouth breathing may produce fatal apnoea. This delay in response disappears at 6/12[87]. The most recent evaluation shows that frequent home visiting and help given to high risk families during the first six months of the baby's life improves the 'at risk' baby's chances of survival[84].

role of general practitioner, clinical medical officer and health visitor

In the United Kingdom, following the registration of the child's birth with the local Registrar, parents receive a medical card and NHS code number for their new baby. They can now register the baby with their family doctor. All births are notified by law within 6 hours of birth by prepaid postcard to the Area Medical Officer (AMO)[88]. There is an additional notification of handicap or deformity by the midwife or health visitor to the AMO for the Office of Population Census and Surveys (OPCS).

The domiciliary midwife will visit all discharges from the maternity hospital up to the tenth day and will take the blood for the PKU test. All babies born in hospital will have had their hips checked for congenital dislocation by the doctor or hospital midwife. If the baby is born at home, the test for congenital dislocation of the hip will have been done by the domiciliary midwife or by the family doctor. Premature infants, on discharge from hospital, are followed up by the midwife specializing in the care of premature babies.

On the tenth day, regular home visits and follow up of the baby and family become the responsibility of the health visitor who should visit all new babies at home on or about the tenth day[89]. Health visitors are specially trained state registered nurses (SRN) with midwifery training who have completed a course in child development and acquired special skills and knowledge in helping the mother and her baby. Health visitors, since 1974, have worked more closely with family doctors whether in health centres, group practice premises or single-handed practices, as do district nurses and domiciliary midwives. But apart from health centres, few facilities are provided for health visitors and their offices are often removed from the practice premises. Some areas have paediatric nurses who nurse sick children at home and work as part of the district nursing service.

In the United Kingdom, preventive medical care, child development and health surveillance, including school health, is still largely carried out by clinical medical officers working with health visitors and school nurses, the senior clinical medical officer being the pivot for the community care of the handicapped child. 10–20% of family doctors run a child development and health surveillance service for the pre-school child in their practices[90]. Family doctors are responsible for the treatment of all acute conditions affecting the child and the family. The Committee on the Child Health Services[15] (the Court Report) recommended that family doctors should carry out surveillance of health and child development, thus combining healing and preventive medicine, as, only in this way will there be full cognizance of potential handicapping conditions. It is reported[91] from a practice in the USA that the incidence of otitis media in the first year of life may be as high as 30%. Liverpool[92] and Edinburgh[93] report an incidence of otitis media in infants of 18% and 16% respectively. In the first seven years of life more than 10% of children consult their family doctor in any one year with otitis media. The incidence of residual deafness varies but the most reliable figure[94] showed that 6% of affected children suffered permanent damage to one or both ears. Many more children suffered transitory hearing loss, a serious deprivation at that period of kinaesthetic and auditory appreciation of sound so vital to the development of language and expressive speech and, in later childhood, a serious handicap at school.

Discovery of handicap or the possibility of handicap in an infant should lead to referral to the paediatrician at the district general hospital for investigation, diagnosis and possibly further assessment at the hospital's Child Development Centre. Every child with a physical handicap and/or delayed development should be referred to a consultant paediatrician as early in life as possible[95]. At the Child Development Centre, a team of specialists in child development – paediatrician, senior clinical medical officer, physiotherapist, speech therapist, orthoptist, psychologist, teacher and social worker – will undertake an assessment of the child's abilities as well as the child's disabilities and undertake a therapeutic and supporting service for the handicapped child and his family. The paediatrician or other consultant involved, such as the otologist, ophthalmologist or paediatric neurologist, will be responsible for the diagnosis and, with the family doctor, any genetic guidance needed by the family and later guidance for the affected child in adolescence or young adulthood.

A designated person, either from the hospital team or the community services, will see the parents and child regularly to give continuing advice and support and ensure that any necessary therapy will be continued, but will not encourage unnecessary treatment. Therapy and teaching may be provided at the hospital centre or by the community services. The latter may be more convenient for the child and the parents. Early special education is now available in a variety of nursery schools whether attached to local infant schools or special schools catering for a variety of handicaps. The latter are more likely to have full time staff or regular visits from physiotherapists, speech therapists, and nurses, with frequent attendance by school medical officers and psychologists. Advice to the Local Education Authority on the need for special education by a handicapped child is the responsibility of the Area Specialist for Child Health. This responsibility is carried out on behalf of the Area Specialist (Child Health) by senior doctors of the school health service and in some cases by senior registrars in paediatrics and consultant paediatricians who may act as school medical officers to the special schools. Close liaison by the hospital paediatric department with family doctors and the school health service to give the best possible care to the handicapped child and his family is necessary.

references

1. Dobbing, J. (1974). The later development of the brain and its vulnerability. In Davis, J. A. and Dobbing, J. (eds.) *The Scientific Foundation of Paediatrics*. (London: Heinemann)
2. Fitzhardings, P.M. and Stevens, E.M. (1972). The small for dates infant. II. Neurological and intellectual sequelae. *J. Paediatr.*, **50**
3. Editoral (1972) Measuring placental function. *Br. Med. J.*, **1**, 193
4. Thompson, E. H., *et al.* (1965). Fetal development as determined by ultrasound pulse echo techniques. *Am. J. Obstet. Gynecol.*, **92**, 44
5. Butler, N. R., Goldstein, H. and Ross, E. M. (1972). Cigarette smoking in pregnancy: its influence on birth weight and perinatal mortality. *Br. Med. J.*, **2**, 127
6. Robertson, N.R.C. and Tizard, J.P.M. (1975). Prognosis for infants with idiopathic respiratory distress syndrome. *Br. Med. J.*, **ii**, 271
7. Rush, R.W. *et al.* (1976). Contribution of pre-term delivery to perinatal mortality. *Br. Med. J.*, **2**, 965
8. Usher, R. and McLean, F. H. (1974). Normal fetal growth and the significance of fetal growth retardation. In Davis, J.A. and Dobbing, J. (eds.). *Scientific Foundations of Paediatrics*. (London:

Heinemann)

9. Damoulaki-Spakianski, E., Robertson, A. and Cordero, L. (1972). Skin creases on the sole of the foot as a physical index of maturity: comparison between Caucasian and Negro infants. *J. Paediatr.*, **50**, 483
10. Dubowitz, L. M. S., Dubowitz, V. and Goldberg, C. (1970). Clinical assessment of gestational age in the newborn infant. *J. Paediatr.*, **77**, 1
11. Robinson, R. J. (1966). Assessment of gestational age by neurological examination. *Arch. Dis. Child.*, **41**, 437
12. Gordon, R. R. (1977). Premature baby statistics. *Br. Med. J.*, **1**, 1313
13. Newcombe, R. and Chalmers, I. (1977). Changes in distribution of gestational age and birth weight among firstborn infants of Cardiff residents. *Br. Med. J.*, **2**, 925
14. Ounsted, M. and Sleigh, G. (1975). The infant's self-regulation of food intake and weight gain. *Lancet*, **1**, 1393
15. Report of the Committee on the Child Health Services (1976). *Fit for the Future*. (London: HMSO)
16. Editorial (1975). What future for perinatal care? *Lancet*. **1**, 1227
17. Health Services Development (1976). *Report of the Working Party on the Prevention of Early Neonatal Mortality and Morbidity*. (London: HMSO)
18. Report on Health and Social Subjects No. 9. (1974). *Present Day Practice in Infant Feeding*. (London: HMSO)
19. Hanson, L. A. (1976). Escherichia coli infections in childhood. *Arch. Dis. Child.*, **51**, 737
20. Shanks, R. A. (1973). Infant feeding. In Forfar, J. D. and Arneil, G. C. (eds.) *A Textbook of Paediatrics*. (Edinburgh: Churchill Livingstone)
21. Addy, D. P. (1976). Infant feeding: a current review. *Br. Med. J.*, **1**, 1268
22. Holzel, A. (1975). Cow's milk allergy. Some clinical and immunological aspects. *Postgrad. Med. J.*, **51**, 71
23. Belton, N. R. *et al.* (1977). Clinical and biochemical assessment of modified evaporated milk for infant feeding. *Arch. Dis. Child.*, **52**, 167
24. Fosbrooke, A. D. and Wharton, B. A. (1975) 'Added lactose' and 'Added sucrose': Cow's milk formulae in nutrition of low birth weight babies. *Arch. Dis. Child.*, **50**, 409
25. City of Cape Town. Annual Report of the Medical Officer of Health, 1974.
26. Bowlby, J. (1971). *Attachment and Loss*. (Harmondsworth: Penguin Books)
27. Editorial (1977). Congenital dislocation of the hip. *Br. Med. J.*, **1**, 1303
28. Von Rosen, S. (1962). Diagnosis and treatment of the congenital

dislocation of the hip joint in the newborn. *J. Bone Jt. Surg.*, **44**B, 284

29. Barlow, T. G. (1962). Early diagnosis and treatment of congenital dislocation of the hip. *J. Bone Jt. Surg.*, **44**B, 292
30. Coleman, S. S. (1956). Diagnosis of congenital dysplasia of the hip in the newborn infant. *J. Am. Med. Assoc.*, **162**, 548
31. Ortolani, M. (1937). Un sego poco noto e sua importanza per la diagnose precoce de prelussazione congenita dell'anca. *Paediatria*, **45**, 129
32. Harrold, A. J. (1977). Problems in congenital dislocation of the hip. *Br. Med. J.*, **1**, 1071
33. Raine, D. N. (1974). Screening for disease: inherited metabolic disease. *Lancet,* **2**, 996
34. Forfar, J. O. (1973). Metabolic Disorders. In Forfar, J. O. and Arneil, G. C. (eds.) *A Textbook of Paediatrics,* (Edinburgh: Churchill Livingstone)
35. World Health Organisation Scientific Group (1968). *Screening for Inborn Errors of Metabolism.* (WHO)
36. Guthrie, R. and Susi, A. (1963). A simple method for detecting phenylketonuria in large populations of newborn infants. *J. Paediatr.,* **32**, 338
37. Scriver, C.R., Davies, E. and Cullen, A.M. (1964). Application of a simple micromethod to the screening of plasma for a variety of aminoacidopathies. *Lancet,* **2**, 230
38. May, E.D. (1977). Parent reaction to medical care and screening. In Raine, D.N. (ed.) *Medico-Social Management of Inherited Metabolic Disease.* (Lancaster: MTP Press)
39. Holt, K.S. (1974). Screening for disease: infancy and childhood. *Lancet,* **2**, 1057
40. Rutter, M. (1974). *Maternal Deprivation Reassessed.* (Harmondsworth: Penguin Books)
41. Minde, K. (1976). Child psychiatry in developing countries. *J. Child Psychol. Psychiatry,* **17**, 79
42. Sheridan, M. D. (1968). *The Developmental Progress of Infants and Young Children.* (London: HMSO)
43. Egan, D., Illingworth, R. S. and MacKeith, R. C. (1969). *Developmental Screening 0–5 years.* (London: Spastics Society and Heinemann)
44. Frankenburg, W. K. and Dodds, J. B. (1967). The Denver developmental screening test. *J. Paediatr.*, **71**, 181
45. Macfarlane, A. (1977). *The Psychology of Childbirth.* (London: Fontana/Open Books)
46. Winnicott, D. W. (1957). *The Child and the Outside World.* (London: Tavistock Publications Ltd.)
47. Karlin, I., David, K. and Guren, L. (1977). *Development and Disorders of Speech in Childhood.* (New York: Thomas)
48. Wolff, P. H. (1967). The role of biological rhythms in early

psychological development. *Bull. Meninger Clin.*, **31**, 197

49. Wolff, P. H. (1969). The natural history of crying and other vocalisations in early infancy. In Foss, B.M. (ed.) *Determinants of Infant Behaviour.* (London: Methuen)
50. Wybar, K. (1974). *Ophthalmology.* (London: Baillière-Tindall)
51. Fantz, R. L. (1966). Pattern discrimination and selective attention as determinants of perceptual development from birth. Kidd, A. H. and Rivoire, J. L. (eds.) *Perceptual Development in Children.* (New York: International Universities Press)
52. Piaget, J. (1955). *The Child's Construction of Reality.* (London: Routledge and Kegan Paul)
53. Schaffer, H. R. (1971). *The Growth of Sociability.* (Harmondsworth: Penguin Books)
54. Schaffer, H. R. and Emerson, P. E. (1964). The development of social attachments in infancy. *Monogr. Soc. Res. Child Devel.*, **29**
55. Ainsworth M. D. S. (1967). *Infancy in Uganda.* (New York: Johns Hopkins Press)
56. Editorial (1977). Screening children for visual defects. *Br. Med. J.*, **2**, 594
57. Griffiths, R. (1954). *The Abilities of Babies.* (London: University of London Press)
58. *Immunisation Programmes for Children: Report of a Working Group with the participation of the International Children's Centre* (1977) (Copenhagen: World Health Organisation)
59. Salimpour, R. (1977). Cause of death in tetanus neonatorum: a study of 233 cases with 54 necropsies. *Arch. Dis. Child.*, **52,** 587
60. Springett, V. H. (1972). Tuberculosis – epidemiology in England and Wales. *Br. Med. J.*, **1**, 422
61. DHSS (1973). *Tuberculosis – Epidemiology and Control.* (London: HMSO)
62. DHSS (1977). *Whooping Cough Vaccination: Review of the Evidence on Whooping Cough Vaccination by the Joint Committee on Vaccination and Immunisation.* (London: HMSO)
63. Harker, P. (1977). Primary immunisation and febrile convulsions in Oxford. *Br. Med. J.*, **2**, 490
64. Salk, J., and Salk, D. (1977). Control of influenza and poliomyelitis with killed virus vaccines. *Science*, **195**, 834
65. Krugman, S., Ward, R. and Katz, S. L. (1977). *Infectious Diseases in Children.* (St. Louis: C. V. Mosby Co.)
66. Cossart, Y. E. (1977). Evolution of poliovirus since the introduction of attenuated vaccine. *Br. Med. J.*, **1**, 1621
67. Nicholas, D. D., Kratzer, J. H., Ofosu-Amaah, S. and Belcher, D. W. (1977). Is poliomyelitis a serious problem in developing countries? – the Danfa experience. *Br. Med. J.*, **1,** 1009
68. Morley, D. (1973). *Medical Priorities in Developing Countries.* (London: Butterworth)
69. Tripp, J. H., Wilmers, M. and Wharton, B.A. (1977). Gastro-

enteritis: a continuing problem of child health in Britain. *Lancet,* **2**, 233
70. White, F. A. (1976). *Widening Horizons of Child Health.* (Lancaster: MTP Press)
71. Registrar-General (1973). *Statistical Review of England and Wales for 1971.* (London: HMSO)
72. Caffey, J. (1946). *Am. J. Roentgenol.*, **56**, 163
73. Woolley, P. V. and Evans, W. A. (1955). *J. Am. Med. Assoc.*, **158**, 539
74. Kempe, C. H., *et al.* (1962). The battered child syndrome. *J. Am. Med. Assoc.*, **181**, 17
75. Kempe, C. H. (1971). Paediatric implications of the battered baby syndrome. *Arch. Dis. Child.,* **46**, 28
76. MacKeith, R. C. (1974). Speculations on non-accidental injury as a cause of chronic brain disorder. *Devel. Med. Child Neurol.,* **16**, 216
77. Editorial (1971). Sudden death in infants. *Lancet,* **2**, 1017
78. Selwyn Smith, M., and Hanson, R. (1974). 134 battered children: a medical and psychological study. *Br. Med. J.,* **2**, 666
79. Harcourt, B. and Hopkins, D. (1971). Ophthalmic manifestations of the battered baby syndrome. *Br. Med. J.,* **2**, 398
80. Mushin, A. S. (1971). Ocular damage in the battered baby syndrome. *Br. Med. J.*, **2**, 402
81. Sheldon, B. (1978). Practice in social work: A re-examination of a tenuous relationship. *Br. J. Soc. Work,* **8**, 1
82. Ministry of Health: Reports on Public Health and Medical Subjects no. 113. (1965). *Enquiry into Sudden Death in Infancy.* (London: HMSO)
83. DHSS Reports on Public Health and Medical Subjects no. 125. (1970). *Confidential Enquiry into Post-neonatal Deaths.* (London: HMSO)
84. Carpenter, R. G., Gardener, A., McWeeney, P. M. and Emery, J. L. (1977). Multistage scoring system for identifying infants at risk of unexpected death. *Arch. Dis. Child.,* **52**, 606
85. Bergman, R. B., Beckwith, J. B. and Ray, C. G. (1970). *High Risk Factors of Prematurity and Low Birth Weight.* (Seattle: University of Washington Press)
86. Valdes-Dapena, M. A. (1967). Sudden and unexpected death in infancy: a review of the world literature. *J. Paediatr.*, **39**, 123
87. Swift, P. G. and Emery, J. L. (1973). Clinical observations on response to nasal occlusion in infancy. *Arch. Dis. Child.,* **48**, 947
88. National Health Service Act (1977). (London: HMSO)
89. The National Health Service (Re-organisation) Act (1973). (London: HMSO)
90. Irvine, D., and Jeffreys, M. (1971). BMA Planning Unit Survey of General Practice, 1969. *Br. Med. J.*, **2**, 535
91. Hoeckelman, R. A. (1977). Infectious illness during the first year

of life. *J. Paediatr.*, **59**, 119
92. Lowe, J. F., Bamforth, J. S. and Pracy, R. (1963). Acute otitis media. One year in general practice. *Lancet,* **2**, 1130
93. Paterson, J. E. and MacLean, D. W. (1970). Acute otitis media in children: a medico-social study from general practice. *Scott. Med. J.*, **15**, 289
94. Neil, J. F., *et al.* (1966). Deafness in acute otitis media. *Br. Med. J.*, **1**, 75
95. Griffiths, M. I. (1973). *The Young Retarded Child.* (London: Churchill Livingstone)

chapter three
the years from 1 to 3

normal motor development

At the beginning of their second year most normal babies will be walking, first with one hand held, then rapidly, alone – apart from a small group, approximately 10%, who shuffle[1]. When shuffling, the baby slides forward on both buttocks or one buttock and a flexed lower limb, described as hitching or scooting in the USA[2]. These infants develop sitting and standing balance later than their peers and have a prolongation of the wide-based toddler gait due to a lag in the maturation of the spinal motor tracts causing hypotonia[3]. This maturation lag affects the trunk and all four limbs but resolves in a cephalo-caudal fashion in 2–3 years. There are no abnormal neurological signs and there is a family history in 50% of cases[3]. The babies particularly dislike being in the prone position and this position should be avoided[4]. It is an important point to remember in giving advice on therapy and positioning for handicapped babies as the infant will not respond, or will be slow to respond, to therapy in the prone position and may be misjudged as retarded or difficult.

normal social and emotional development

Social and emotional development depends upon the temperament with which we are born and the environmental influences of home, school and society generally. A longitudinal study[5] of behaviour and temperament shows a persistence of qualities evident from early infancy; the baby who wriggles during nappy changing will be into everything as a toddler, the quiet baby will be a quiet five-year-old. These qualities appear to be independent of the personality of the parents and the way they handle their children.

Toddlers, from about 13 months of age, are able to show spontaneous affection towards their parents and other children. By 18 months they are also able to express anger and will do so by hitting and pulling but with little hostility in the action. They may have temper tantrums[6]. Jealousy will also be expressed and particularly worries parents when shown towards a new baby in the family although the parents, quite correctly, give more attention than usual to the toddler. The jealousy is due to the young child's inability to understand the situation as he sees the new baby receiving his parents' attention, therefore thinking that he has a rival for their affection and attention.

By the time they reach their second birthday, children can experience a wide range of emotions and may have developed fears of the dark or being alone[6]. Although many fears will be alleviated in the process of growing up, the real depth and intensity of small children's fears and anger are probably underestimated by most adults. The basis of mental and sexual health is laid down in infancy and childhood, as are the aberrations and abnormalities experienced by adults[7]. An understanding of children's loves and fears and the need to express these in play and fantasy is necessary for the normal adult development.

Children need to be loved and able to express their love towards their fathers and mothers. A warm loving relationship between parents and children is more effective in developing acceptable behaviour than the use of parental disapproval. Immature parents may have difficulty in giving warmth and comfort to their children as was seen when a 2-year-old hit his head in the children's clinic while his mother was discussing her own emotional problems. Although the child cried bitterly, his mother made no attempt to comfort him. The doctor had to pick the child up and put him on his mother's knees and place her arms about the child before the mother gave her child the attention and comfort he needed when he quietened immediately.

Children under two years of age cannot relate socially with others of the peer group apart from an awareness of their presence and will only play alongside other children in parallel play by 3 years of age[6]. Play with other children, apart from siblings, is an important landmark in social development and is dependent on the ability of the child to communicate through speech and language.

sleep

'The need for discipline or habit-training and security as a base for adventure is not always appreciated, but in my view all properly conducted adventures must have a base of security, and the adventure of childhood is no exception.'[8] The importance of regular bedtime as a habit in childhood cannot be overstated. Parents need to control the amount of exciting play, television and stimulating drinks such as tea and coffee before bedtime. It is surprising how early in childhood some children are introduced to tea and coffee and enquiry about the type of drink offered to children who present with sleep disorders is an essential part of history taking.

Children vary in their need for sleep and after the first year of life need on average ten hours in any 24 hours. Length of sleep is determined by changes in growth development and will be affected by anxieties and fears. Children need to be warm and comfortable and, if fearful of the dark, should be given a soft night light. A quiet period before going to bed, a warm drink and a warm bath will help children to relax and encourage sleep. Rituals that are important to the child need to be observed as they lessen anxiety whether the ritual is a bedtime story, prayers or potting Teddy.

mealtimes

Regular mealtimes are also important although the amount of food required may be regulated by the child. A study[9] of the nutrition of children between the ages of 6 months and 4½ years showed that, although milk was the most important source of food for the youngest children, by 18 months of age the diet of all children included most of the foods used in the adult mixed diet. The management of fads requires sympathetic support for parents but fads like tastes should be tolerated and not made a battlefield between the parents and the child. As Apley and MacKeith[10] suggest, 'Parents hope their chil-children will become adults with discriminating tastes in all fields; it seems reasonable to treat these preferences with respect . . . It should be made easy for the child to resume eating without losing face.'

developmental problems of ethnic minorities

In any multi-racial society, one has to temper judgement of what is normal in relation to the developmental experience of children of different ethnic origins. Serious deprivation is more likely to occur when both parents work and the child is minded by unsuitable people. This happens more frequently in West Indian and African families and affects their children's speech and language development more than their motor skills[11]. Many mothers in the Asian community are now working in cottage industries and factories, causing their children privation of language and play, and the necessity of being bilingual. Itinerant caravan dwelling 'travellers' tend not to provide their children with toys and play material[12].

Children in Asian and travellers' families are bottle-fed for longer periods than usual, up to 18 months or two years and sometimes longer to prevent messy feeding. Asian families tend to eat with their fingers, and in these groups children may not know what forks and spoons are. These and their use are common items in screening language and social behaviour. Similar problems may arise with chairs, as Asian families eat sitting on the floor and travellers have fixed seating in their caravans. A most memorable sight was a delightful, plump, Asian lady, dressed in bright yellow satin trousers, trying to demonstrate in mime that her son appeared unable to squat on the floor for his meals. In her excitement the dear lady took off in a glorious slide on her bottom across the room, whereupon her son and the doctor became convulsed with laughter, her son proving conclusively that he could squat. His mother, quite unhurt, sportingly joined in the general fun. Physical examination confirmed that there was no abnormality and further information proved that the boy preferred to sit in the family's only armchair at mealtimes to be waited on by his sisters.

Manual dexterity was noticeably poor in mothers and children amongst a group of Irish tinkers. These mothers no longer make craft articles nor do they knit or sew, and they found holding a pen difficult[12]. Mothers in minority ethnic groups are often illiterate and have poor linguistic skills[13]. Children of immigrant families may have to learn two languages and, although understanding both languages, may have difficulty in expressing themselves. This delay in developing English language may be misinterpreted.

A sixteen-month-old Asian baby was seen at the request of the health visitor who had reported that the baby was slow and always found sitting in a corner without toys. The father came with the baby to the clinic. He worked in another town but was the only member of the household who spoke English. The father said that his son was normal and that his wife had reassured him that this was so. It became clear that the baby disliked being handled and cried persistently unless left sitting on the floor. The infant was small and unable to stand alone but showed no stigmata of subnormality. He showed no response to sound unless the sound was very loud. The infant's profound hearing loss was confirmed by the consultant otologist. The pre-school teacher of the deaf, with an interpreter, visited the mother and the infant at home to help with the use of the hearing aid and to teach the mother how to speak to her baby. It appears that the baby's inability to respond to his mother, coupled with her loneliness, led the mother to resent and reject her son and to pretend to her husband that their son was normal.

Feelings of resentment in these situations take many years to resolve and, in this case, early admission to a school for deaf children was necessary to help the child. The special problems of mothers who have handicapped children and whose husbands work away from home were reported[14] in 1948. The profoundly deaf child in an Asian family, even with the help of amplification of hearing by aids, is only going to learn one language, preferably the language of the country in which the child is going to reside, and for children brought up in the United Kingdom that language must be English. As most of these children's mothers do not speak English, it is a difficult concept for them to accept.

Toilet training was slow in travellers' children as their mothers work in the fields and do not have time to potty their children, but incontinence is not a noticeable problem among the children of immigrant parents[12].

perceptual development

We develop visual perception by seeing and perceiving objects and shapes and recognizing their variation in relation to each other, the environment and distance. Perception enables us to act appropriately in our environment and to feel secure in controlling our environment. Human perception depends on memory and the close involvement of language[15]. In the pre-verbal infant and children who are deaf, speech impaired or severely mentally handicapped, memory storage is probably by images rather than words.

The internal image of the body's position in space and the relationship between the body parts is maintained by the parietal lobes, which control the direction of gaze, visual attention and perception and the skilled co-ordination of eye-hand movements[16]. Severing the connections between the parietal lobes by section of the corpus callosum destroys the unity of body image. Disorders of visual perception and visual attention may follow lesions in the parietal cortex. In adults, parietal lobe lesions cause an alteration in the perception of body form and its relation to space with an inability to direct visual attention to the contralateral field. This is accompanied by slowness or lack of volition in achieving fixation of gaze on objects and difficulty in disengaging fixation although eye movements are full – oculomotor apraxia[17]. There is no oculomotor paralysis.

Learning about variations in size and shape caused by aspect and distance is initiated in the first year of life by the infant throwing toys and objects from the pram and the high-chair, and, on an increasing scale, by the toddler in exploration of the environment. The toddler with the development of expressive speech learns to name an object or to make a sound imitating the name of an object and discovers that his mother will give him the object. The discovery of names, followed by the discovery of the characteristics and the function of objects, is the early development of concept formation. Young children perceive whole objects rather than details and recognize objects as easily when they are presented upside down, and they make no distinction between left and right. With increasing mobility, the toddler will compare new objects with previous experience and learn to predict the behaviour of an object and how to react to it. With speech and language development the child learns to actively modify the stimuli acting upon him and to adapt his behaviour to these modifications thus learning to control his environment[18].

The development of attention occurs first in response to adult direction and it is not until a child learns to speak and can name an object for himself that he can distinguish it from other objects and so direct his attention voluntarily to it. Direction of attention to a named object can only take place in a young child if there are no distractions. The formation of an efficient and stable form of voluntary attention does not develop until shortly before a child's fifth birthday[18].

language development

The four basic language skills are listening, speaking, reading and writing, often divided into comprehension and expression, comprehension always preceding expression[13].

Listening and comprehension are dependent on an intact auditory and visual pathway. We need to see lip movements and gestures as well as facial expression to listen: so correction of refractive errors is important to the normal hearing and to the hearing handicapped.

During the second year, development of social and language skills are most noticeable, from single words at the end of infancy to two to three word combinations at 18 months, e.g. 'me go', 'drink now', and, by 3 years of age, the child will be using six syllable sentences such as 'I have a little cat' and will be able to name small toys when requested to do so.

Delayed language development, with or without speech disorder and more marked than tests of non-verbal intelligence would suggest, is one of the most common problems in young children in some areas of Britain today. The estimated incidence[19] of severe disorder in children is 1 : 1000, whilst a survey[20] of three-year-olds in Newcastle-upon-Tyne showed 6% to have delayed language and 11% unintelligible speech.

The common perinatal factors in a group of speech defective children[21] were:

(1) Premature delivery, i.e. less than 37 weeks,

(2) 50% more boys than girls,

(3) 4th or later children in large families, and

(4) Social class 4 and 5.

In this group, the speech defective children were more likely to be clumsy, to have refractive errors and squints and to be maladjusted on the Bristol Social Adjustment Guide[22].

Many studies have shown that children in large families,

isolated communities and homes with inadequate intellectual stimulation may grow up with seriously retarded verbal abilities which are more noticeable as the children get older suggesting progressive impairment due to a lack of stimulation – a privation of communication between parent and child rather than a deprivation meaning loss of communication[23]. It is a common fallacy that children learn language from each other. This is not true. They learn language from the adults around them.

One of the best classifications of speech disorder is that of Ingram[24] (table 6).

Once experienced in the normal development of infants and young children, one should never be afraid to question the results from the most illustrious second opinion if they do not accord with subsequent findings, such as the child with speech or language delay or behaviour disorder, said to have passed his hearing tests, yet who appears to be deaf. Hearing tests should be repeated and the child referred back to the consultant if there is any doubt about the result. Intelligent children will gain clues from all sorts of sources such as reflections of movement in the glasses of the operator, their parents' muscle tone and held breath. Older schoolchildren with vision defects have been known to memorize the eye chart while the tester is distracted by their school friends so that they can read it accurately from memory at 6 metres. Intelligent children with handicaps are often the most difficult to assess and the most rewarding to unravel. We need to use all the expertise available in medicine, psychology and education. A very intelligent boy with seriously delayed speech and language development gave inconclusive results to hearing testing between 18/12 and 3 years, including a trial with a hearing aid supervised by a teacher of the deaf. He was under the care of an experienced otologist, and consistent results, confirming a high tone hearing loss of the order of 80–90 dB, were only obtained after daily observation and assessment. Once diagnosis was made, correct prescription of hearing aids and admission to a unit for partially hearing children meant improved hearing ability and rapid development in his speech and language.

Having excluded major sensory handicap and severe mental handicap as a cause of speech and language delay, one should be aware of the possibility of severe psychological disorder such as autism. The incidence of autism is estimated

table 6

classification of speech disorders

(1)	*Dysphonia*	–	a disorder of voicing, an abnormal volume of sound
(2)	*Dysrhythmia*	–	a disorder of co-ordination of articulation, e.g. stuttering or stammering.
(3)	*Dysarthria*	–	difficulty in speaking due to a structural abnormality, which may be either: (a) neurological – an upper or lower motor neuron lesion. (b) physical – abnormality of the palate, tongue, lips, jaw, etc.
(4)	*Secondary speech disorders*	–	(a) mental retardation (b) deafness (c) true dysphasia (d) psychiatric, e.g. autism (e) environmental
(5)	*Specific developmental speech disorders*	–	In the mild and moderate forms, comprehension is normal, acquisition of expressive speech is slow, and articulation may be infantile. In the more severe forms, comprehension is retarded or absent such as in central auditory imperception and expressive speech either severely retarded or absent.

as 2–4/10 000 children and, if it is suspected, a useful questionnaire is that produced by Dr Lorna Wing[25] from the features of childhood autism as outlined by Creak and Kanner. Autistic children either do not develop language or, if expressive speech is present, it is not used to communicate with family and friends. Echolalia, either immediate or delayed, is often present. The affected children appear to be unable to relate to people and situations and avoid emotional contact, noticeably by gaze avoidance. This is often associated with aimless repetitive motor movement of hands or body, e.g. hand flapping as in blind children and pirouetting.

Expressive aphasia due to severe deprivation should be kept in mind. This is not elective mutism. Paul was referred by the health visitor at 2½ years with delayed speech development. He had passed his hearing test at 8/12. Paul was impossible to examine as he was so mobile and overactive. Motor development, head circumference, eardrums and eye movements appeared normal and he was physically fit. Paul's overactivity was in complete contrast to his mother's almost total immobility – a perfect representation of flat affect. She was a chronic schizophrenic living in a single upstairs room. Three older children were in the care of the local authority and, apart from Paul, there were twins aged 8/12 at home. Paul was penned in the twins' cot all day. Although Paul had no idea how to play and merely grabbed every toy or ball presented to him, trying to hide them, he showed flashes of humour and could be playful momentarily. He did not appear to be unintelligent. Further hearing testing at a specialist clinic showed no evidence of hearing loss. Paul attended the hospital assessment centre, where physical examination including motor development and vision was found to be normal. He was continent and was of normal intelligence on performance testing. Paul's aphasia was due to gross deprivation. He and the twins were admitted urgently to a local day nursery, with the support of an experienced speech therapist. At 7 years, his speech sounds are normal but his language development is retarded. He has proved to be an intelligent boy and has coped in the infant department (age range 5–7 years) of his local school with continuing support from the speech therapist and the educational psychologist. However, Paul will need a special unit providing a smaller class and individual help at junior school (age range 8–11 years) when a more complex language structure, reading and writing will create problems and possibly severe stresses on his limited language development, particularly with such an unsupportive home background. The twins' speech and language development appears to be progressing in a normal but slow pattern.

Imitative play as a measure of the inner language (comprehension) of young children may give important clues to intelligence and the presence or absence of sensory handicap. A five-year-old boy, reported to be mentally handicapped, was playing with the toys while his mother was being interviewed. The boy picked up the toy telephone and mimed a telephone conversation perfectly with lip movements and facial expression but quite silently. His intelligence was in the normal range on performance testing and his high tone hearing loss was confirmed by the otologist. Unfortunately, the boy's deafness was complicated by a central language disorder and his development of speech appears to be permanently frustrated.

behaviour disorder

When a child presents with a behaviour disorder, handicap should be excluded for, if present, explanation given to the parents will often alleviate stress and anxiety. In the case illustrated, the mother had successfully avoided the specialists who were best able to help her understand her son's handicap. The health visitor and family doctor eventually persuaded the mother to attend with her son to see the senior clinical medical officer at the local clinic.

The history showed an unhappy pregnancy complicated by pre-eclampsia, followed by a difficult delivery. The child, John, had had an equally stormy infancy with a fractured skull at 8 months of age. Investigation proved that this injury was not the result of battering, although his parents were unmarried and the cohabitation was unsettled and prone to outbreaks of violence. Prior to the clinic visit, John's parents had separated and he and his mother were now living in a flat with his mother's sister.

John's mother was bitter and angry with the doctor. She refused to allow John to undress for the examination and when persuaded to remove his topcoat she did so with such ferocity the child cried. Peace was restored by persuading the mother to sit and allowing John to sit on her knee. At the desk, John was introduced to the toys and was playing happily until his mother gradually pulled him away so that he could not reach the toys. John then kicked his mother on the shin and was allowed to play on the floor.

John, then aged 4 years, was an apparently bright boy with good language development. His speech was clear and, although his mother would not allow formal examination, it was noticed that John's glasses were clear and he was wearing a patch. At the desk he had difficulty in seeing small toys and an obvious nystagmus. Playing on the floor, John again showed difficulty in seeing small objects and was unable to see a dark red ball the size of a tennis ball on the multi-coloured carpet.

John's mother relaxed somewhat and talked about her fears and problems. Their home was an upstairs flat with a downstairs toilet. John had frequent falls on the poorly lighted staircase resulting in frequent bruising. His mother was fearful she would be accused of battering him and so she encouraged John's bad behaviour to avoid examination or failed to keep appointments. On contacting the eye hospital, it was confirmed that either appointments had been failed or John had been so naughty that attempts at refraction had to be abandoned.

When John's mother understood that his many falls on the stairs and elsewhere were due to his poor eyesight as well as poor lighting she promised to keep an appointment with the eye specialist. She had presumed that as he had glasses and a patch, no further treatment was necessary. John's mother refused to accept that he would have any problems at school, either with his vision or his behaviour. Rehousing was also refused.

John was refracted and, with his new glasses, he improved

socially and emotionally. As a rising five, he was admitted to the local infant's school but sent home that same day. The continuation of his violent behaviour and poor eyesight was too great a problem for his class teacher and his school. His mother then agreed to visit the local school for the visually handicapped child and was delighted when she saw what a pleasant place it was. For the first few months at his special school, John's behaviour was frightful but, in a small class with excellent teachers and with a more tranquil parent, he settled. At 8 years of age, he is a lively intelligent boy ready to leave his special school and to go to his local school. John's mother has made a happy marriage so the longterm prognosis is hopeful.

preventive medicine

measles vaccination

Following the course of triple antigen and oral polio immunization, i.e. primary immunization during the baby's first year, one injection of live attenuated measles virus should be given after 13 months of age and at least one month after completing the primary course of immunization. The vaccine can be administered up to 15 years of age. The child's antibody response to measles vaccine was found to be 92% in babies immunized at 13 months and only 67% if immunization was carried out when the baby is under 12 months of age, with a consequent higher clinical attack rate[26].

Measles vaccine must always be handled as recommended by the manufacturers, before and after reconstitution, with checks on refrigeration and exposure to light. When a child, who was thought to be immunized, has had a severe attack of measles, it has been found[27] that either the child was not immunized, one of the less reliable early programmes and vaccines had been used or the vaccine had lost its antigenicity, either through poor refrigeration or exposure to light.

Follow up[28] of 5000 children immunized in 1964 in a Medical Research Council trial with live attenuated measles virus (Schwartz strain) or killed vaccine followed by live vaccine (Enders–Edmonston B strain) showed no waning of protection in either group after 12 years, although protection was better in the early years with the live vaccine. In the same trial it was shown that the attack rate in an unvaccinated, highly exposed group was ten times that in the vaccinated group. When measles occurred in immunized children, the cases were milder and required less medical attention. No child in the immunized group needed admission to hospital. It is sad to report that although in 1968 800000 children were immunized in the United Kingdom, in 1975 only 300000 children were immunized[29], and, in the USA, a third of 1–4 year-olds have not been immunized[30], when we know that in an epidemic of measles one patient in 15 has a potentially serious complication and one in a 1000 cases develops measles encephalitis[31].

In tropical countries, measles is often severe especially when a dark, desquamating rash appears[32]. A recent report[33] of measles occurring in 30 malnourished children in Zaria, Nigeria, showed a mortality of 50% and a prolonged morbidity in the survivors. A continuing low rate of measles immunization will mean a higher proportion of susceptible children, susceptible adolescents and susceptible young adults. In the MRC trial[28], 37 unvaccinated children in the 10–12 age group had no detectable level of antibody. The same trial confirmed the persistence of protection after 10 years by serological findings, and Buynak[34] in the USA produced similar findings 14 years after immunization, providing serological evidence of continuing immunity. In the German Democratic Republic, intense immunization campaigns have reduced the incidence[35] of measles from 55633 cases in 1965 to 398 cases in 1974.

dental care

Children should be able to grow up with sound teeth, good occlusion and healthy supporting tissues[36]. Caries is a major dental problem often associated with gingivitis. It is largely due to a high intake of refined carbohydrate in the form of refined sugar and, as mentioned in Chapter 2, sweet drinks in comforters are often the precursors of children's fondness for sugary substances leading to associated dental decay. Early encouragement should be given to children to brush gums and teeth, especially before going to bed. A surprising number of children, when toddlers, are given a biscuit to eat (suck) or a sweet milk drink on going to bed. If a child is thirsty, water is preferable. A soft brush is important – hard nylon may hurt tender gums and the child will then refuse to use a brush. At home and at school, children should be encouraged to rinse their mouths out with water after eating sweets if there is no opportunity for brushing teeth. Brushing teeth does not affect decay but makes a significant contribution to healthy gums[37].

Parents should be encouraged to take their children to the dentist during the child's second year. This will help to allay the children's fears. At present, 30% of children attend the dentist for the first time with toothache, which often means an extraction complicated by the need for a general anaesthetic. A pale, tired six-year-old seen at a routine school medical had a broken infected lower molar ulcerating the mucosal surface of her cheek. This was shown to her mother who explained that she knew but was waiting for the dentist to visit the school, although there was a regular dental session for children at the local clinic. When the importance of treatment was explained to her, the mother took her daughter to the

table 7

drop in dental treatment after fluoridation in the Birmingham Area Health Authority

	1964	*1976*
deciduous teeth extracted in children 0–15 years	44 410	13 813
permanent teeth extracted in children 0–15 years	13 429	6 217
general anaesthetics for dental treatment	1 889	559

clinic the same day for treatment. This was not deliberate neglect but a needy reminder to jog a parent into action. Many parents in Britain have a laisser-faire attitude to dental care and treatment.

Handicapped children also need regular dental attention. This is often neglected especially in the disturbed or behaviour-disordered handicapped child. Whilst so neglected, the presence of serious dental disease may be making the child's behaviour more unmanageable. Regular inspection by doctors and nurses, as well as dentists, of all children will ensure that gross disease is recognized and treated. Handicapped children are more likely to need a general anaesthetic for treatment and, in some cases, for inspection of their teeth. In general, specialist treatment of this nature will be carried out in a hospital dental department.

The best public health measure is undoubtedly fluoridation of the drinking water supply[38,39]. Fluoridation reduces the incidence of caries in children substantially. In the Birmingham Area Health Authority, extractions and general anaesthetics in children's dental clinics showed a marked drop after the water supply was fluoridated in 1964 (table 7). Children who have regular dental treatment, and therefore less current decay, do not have less disease unless there is a source of fluoride to reduce caries[40].

accidents, poisonings and injury

accidents and injury

In 1971, 4651 children in the United Kingdom in the 0–4 age group were admitted to hospital with burns and scalds and 100 children died[41]. Two fifths of fatal accidents occur in and around the home, bad design of housing being the chief cause. Britain has the worst record in Europe for road traffic accidents to child pedestrians[42]. This is not surprising when it has been shown[43] that 19% of mothers thought it safe to allow their 2-year-old children to cross a busy road without supervision. In the USA, it is believed that for every fatal accident to a child, 100–200 non-fatal accidents occur and 1 in 40 of these results in permanent disability[44]. The factors that are most commonly associated with road traffic accidents are:

(1) Bad training and example – the parents who won't use a pedestrian crossing, who cross the road at red traffic lights even with quite small children in tow, and who do not dress their children to be seen in periods of poor visibility.

(2) Bad road-planning and engineering which makes periods of poor visibility more dangerous.

(3) Drivers overestimating children's ability in traffic.

(4) Associated handicap in the child, especially those handicaps involving hearing and vision. A child with an arrested hydrocephalus and an unrecognized partial optic atrophy was knocked down by a car the first time he was allowed to go to school by himself. It is important to explain to parents how seriously handicapped a child with high myopia is on crossing the road if his glasses are missing or broken.

poisonings

Poisoning in childhood reflects standards of living as well as local customs and whether children live in a rural or urban community. Medicines and household cleaning agents are common causes of poisoning in urban communities whereas pesticides are common in rural communities. Paraffin in India, where it is used for heating, is responsible for 40% of cases of accidental poisoning in childhood and, in the USA, pesticides are now responsible for more deaths in children under 4 years than all other substances[45]. Seasonal plants may result in poisoning, the most common in Britain being laburnum seeds. Early treatment of poisoning by induced vomiting to remove the poisonous material should be tried. Tickling the back of the throat or giving syrup of ipecacuanha is more effective than gastric lavage. Syrup of ipecacuanha caused emesis[46] in 98% of cases in a series reported by the Salt Lake City Control Center. Salt and water should not be used as an emetic as it may cause hypernatraemia and death[47]. Children who have taken overdoses of medicines or poisonous material should be admitted to hospital for observation.

drowning

Drowning is the third most common cause of death between 1 and 4 years in the USA[48], and accounts for over half the accidental deaths to boys in Finland[41]. The sequence of events in drowning can be divided into four stages:

(1) Primary apnoea during which the glottis is closed.

(2) Dyspnoea with struggling and finally loss of consciousness.

(3) Terminal apnoea with gradual loss of reflexes and a fall in blood pressure.

(4) Cardiac arrest.

When an apparently drowned child is pulled from the water, the mouth should be cleared of debris and vomit and artificial ventilation, using mouth to mouth resuscitation, given. As soon as the equipment is available, intubation and suction can be employed. This equipment is usually available in special schools with swimming baths. In fresh water drowning, haemodilution with hyponatraemia will occur. In salt water drowning, haemoconcentration will arise. If there is cardiac arrest, external cardiac massage should be given at 60 compressions per minute with a breath every fifth compression by the expired-air method. Resuscitation should be continued until there is unequivocal evidence of death, e.g. a flat EEG.

Hypothermia is the important problem in drowning as the main danger to life is cold or a combination of cold and drowning[49]. Severe hypothermia should be distinguished from cardiac arrest as the treatment is different. If a child is conscious when rescued, he is unlikely to have severe hypothermia. As his core temperature falls due to heat loss on rescue the child may lose consciousness rapidly. Severe hypothermia is likely to be present if a body is in a life jacket and found apparently dead. The child should be handled as little as possible, the most urgent problem being to warm him. Wet clothes are removed and the child placed in a bath of warm (hand hot) water keeping the arms and the legs out of the bath water. The best method of central rewarming is to make the patient breathe hot, moist air or oxygen[48]. If deterioration occurs in the bath, ventricular fibrillation is likely. If ventricular fibrillation is present, cardiac massage is applied with artificial ventilation at half the usual rate (30–40 thrusts per minute in the sternum and 10 breaths per minute).

burns

Fire and matches are fascinating to children and they need to learn about the use and the dangers of fire and heat without experiencing the trauma of being burned. Children need to understand the wider dangers of fire to their community and to animal and plant life when fire destroys property and woodland.

Most cases of burns occur in the home when children are alone. Severe scarring of the face and the chest is likely when a small child is able to pull a hot kettle or saucepan on top of himself. Flammable clothing, especially girls' nightdresses and evening gowns, is a source of serious burns to the body when open fires are left unguarded. Pyjamas, the use of non-inflammable material for garments, and fixed fireguards that remain in situ will reduce the number of such accidents.

Simple scalds or burns with intact skin should be immersed in cold water for a few seconds and covered with a sterile dry dressing. If the burnt child is shocked or there is a large burnt area, the burn should be covered with a dry, sterile dressing and the child sent to hospital, preferably to a specialist burns unit. If a sterile dressing is not available, a clean dry cloth may be used. Eyes with chemical burns should be washed with the lids open and irrigated with clean water, the patient being sent to hospital, preferably one with an ophthalmic unit. If possible washing of the eyes should be continued throughout the journey to the hospital.

When the scars of burns are noted on routine examination of children, the history of the accident should be recorded. Occasionally parents unthinkingly encourage their children to believe that a burn or scald acquired as a toddler was the child's fault and this should be recorded. At the school leaving examination the previous history of the burn or scald is discussed and without undermining the child's love and affection for his parents he is gently helped to realize that no toddler or young child could be responsible for such an accident. Hopefully this will prevent the same type of accident in the next generation. Adolescents are always grateful for the help given in understanding their scars. The serious psychological trauma which results from burns and scalds, four out of five children being emotionally disturbed up to five years after the accident, makes every effort in prevention worthwhile.

Accident rates are higher for boys than girls at all ages and boys have a higher mortality rate[50]. In the period 1962–71 the deaths from accidents were 7579 boys and 5179 girls. The death rate for children in social class 5 is twice that for social class 1 – the commonest causes being accidents, respiratory disease, measles and meningococcal infection[51].

The need for adventure and exploration is an essential part of growing up at all stages of childhood – facilities for adventure, preferably with wilderness, which are naturally available for children in rural areas, should be made available for children in urban areas. Children must take some risks in their adventure through childhood and their parents should be encouraged to allow them to do so without foolhardiness.

where should I go?

stay at home

After infancy, children start to move into a different relationship with their parents. From a close direct relationship of great dependence with the mother, the toddler's horizon widens into a triangular relationship, including the father and leading to first steps on the road to maturity[7]. At the same time, parental pressure and expectation for children to become socially competent, e.g. in using a potty, contrasts with their child's experience and enjoyment of self-will. Failure by parents to relieve their baby's thirst or hunger in the first year of life may produce primary anxiety; in the succeeding year, failure of the child to attain or maintain their parents' expectations, as in feeding and becoming continent, will produce anxiety in the child in the form of shame or doubt[52].

Young children are better cared for, get more individual attention and stimulation and are at less risk from infection if they are able to remain at home with their parents. Where the relationship between the parents and between the parents and the child is normal, the home environment is the ideal environment for the child, and gives happiness and contentment to the child and parents[7]. The importance of play for the small child to act out and express fears and hopes must be stressed, especially at this stage of limited verbal expression.

As described in the preceding section on language development, the large family and intellectually deprived environment retards a child's cognitive development and later development of verbal expression. This is especially noticeable where the mother suffers from prolonged depression, either a severe postpuerperal psychosis or the less severe, but no less chronic, form of postpartum depression, perhaps better described as 'the miseries'. The latter is said[53] to occur in 10% of postpartum women, and, in 4%, symptoms were present a year later. Although there is an increased risk of severe depression where there is a preceding history of psychotic breakdown, it is not possible to predict who will be affected in the puerperium[54]. Recent surveys[55,56] found the incidence of depression to be 26–40% in London boroughs, the highest rates occurring in working class women with a child under six years. Four factors increase vulnerability:

(1) Inability to confide in husband or boyfriend.

(2) Not going out to work.

(3) Having been motherless before the age of 11 years.

(4) Having 3 or more children under the age of 14 years.

These families are often housed unsatisfactorily in tower blocks of flats, have less material resources, the mother may be mentally handicapped and the family is often designated a problem family. Rehousing with frequent moves is a ploy used to remove many of these intractable problems, escalating the difficulties under which the children grow up as they lose the neighbours who tolerate them and the professionals in various services (teachers, psychologists, doctors and nurses) who know them and understand their needs.

The association of behaviour disorders in children and adolescents due to emotional and environmental privation at home is well recognized[57,58]. A study in Uganda[59] showed similar findings – broken homes, poverty and frequent moves are commonly associated with maladjustment in children. The questionnaire composed by Rutter[60] is reported to have strong transcultural relevance.

day nursery, day care, playgroup, childminders and crêches

It has been suggested[61] that mothers who want to work should have provision made for the care of their children, the most common form being day nurseries or crêches. Many parents need some relief from the care of their children to maintain their mental health and composure. Some time for babies in a day nursery or a playgroup is thought[62], not only to aid a mother's recovery from postpartum depression, but also to prevent mothers from becoming depressed.

Day nurseries in Britain are run by the Social Services Department and are staffed by nursery nurses. The senior member of staff is called the Officer-in-Charge. Day nurseries accept children from 6/52 to 5 years of age. A fee is charged but this may be waived or staggered in the case of parents who are ill, unemployed or on low earnings. The nurseries are open from 7.30 am to 6.00 pm. Recommendations for admission are arranged through the Area Social Services manager. Priority is given to children thought to be disadvantaged and children of single parent families. Many day nurseries will take handicapped children up to 10% of their numbers. This is probably the right proportion as handicapped children do need extra care and attention.

Nurseries must be staffed adequately if they are to provide proper nurture for young children and not just be a place of relief for parents. An adequate level of perceptual stimulation is necessary for normal psychological functioning as deprivation will lead to poverty of problem solving skills, delayed social development and inappropriate emotional reactions[62]. Residential nurseries take infants and children up to 5–7 years of age for short or long stay care. If the children remain in care after this age they will transfer to children's homes, foster homes or are adopted. The latter two are the preferred form of care. Foster homes are also used for children of all ages whether they are in care for a short or long period of time.

Two groups of handicapped children must be carefully considered before being recommended for admission to day nurseries – children with sensory handicaps, i.e. vision and hearing, and children with severe delay in expressive speech or deviant language development. These handicaps require highly skilled teaching or speech therapy with psychological assessment and review. Most local education authorities will or should have peripatetic teachers for the young blind and deaf child. In the United Kingdom, the Royal National Institute for the Blind (RNIB) also run an education advisory service as most schools for the blind are managed by this organization in contradistinction to schools for the partially sighted which are managed by the local education authorities. The RNIB's education advisors (who are trained teachers of the blind) work very closely with local education authority peripatetic teachers of visually handicapped children and are always willing to see a child and parents.

Pre-school and school services for the profoundly deaf are usually maintained by local education authorities though the Royal National Institute for the Deaf (RNID) do maintain some schools. Early education for the deaf child is well established and most day schools have a nursery department taking children from the age of two years. Teaching by the peripatetic teaching service and parent guidance should start in the first year.

Severe speech and language disorders need the skills of

speech therapists who work very closely with psychologists and teachers advising the children's parents about their development and providing therapy. Again, nursery education should be available and the local education authority has a duty to provide it. The team of speech therapist, psychologist and teachér may be found working from the hospital child development centre or from the community child health and child guidance clinics run by the Health and Education Authorities. Regular follow-up by the doctor and health visitor or school nurse, and liaison with the other professionals is necessary.

day care

Day care centres may be run by the Social Services Department or voluntary societies such as the National Society for the Prevention of Cruelty to Children, Dr. Barnado's or National Children's Homes. They accept children who are known to be disadvantaged (parents who are mentally ill, mentally handicapped or inadequate), children injured by their parents or at risk of injury by their parents and children with known handicaps. Day care centres will have more professional staff such as nursery nurses, teachers, social workers and more frequent visits by doctors, health visitors and psychologists. The children may be escorted from home by car or minibus, when their parents are not able to take them, to the centre and they may be given all their meals at the centre. The children's parents are encouraged to take part in the learning and development of their children and are more closely involved with the staff than in day nurseries. As the social services department pay the fees, even in those centres run by the voluntary societies, the children are only admitted on the recommendation of a social worker.

playgroups

The Pre-School Playgroups Association started in 1961 to provide play for small children and support and respite for their mothers. In 1972, there were 11 500 premises registered providing 280000 places[63]. The playgroup must be registered with the Local Authority under the Nursery and Child Minders Act[64], and will be run by a supervisor and helpers working on a rota basis who may or may not be the mothers of the children attending. A fee is charged. The playgroup philosophy is to concentrate on play as therapy for small children often living confined dreary lives and to encourage development of language and speech. Playgroups can be especially helpful to young mothers of first babies who will sometimes find it easier to confide their problems to the supervisor at the playgroup than to outside professionals such as the health visitor and family doctor. The playgroup may function in various premises including private homes.

child minders

Child minders are women who take children into their homes during the day for varying periods of time. In the United Kingdom, by law[64] they must register with the local social services department. The minders charge a fee and their premises are inspected by the social services department. Despite the scandalous level of care, small children being left in cots all day with no stimulation and very little care, provided by some child minders, often unregistered, the important part played by the many excellent child minders has been recognized. They are fulfilling a need for working mothers which has not been met by other services. Various courses in play and child development are now run in further education establishments and the BBC has screened an imaginative television series using known child minders and describing child development and play. Groups of child minders are now encouraged to work closely with the local day nursery staff.

The conditions and care provided by nurseries and child minders are governed by the Nursery and Childminders Act of 1948[64]. There are still large numbers of unregistered child minders in urban areas, not all bad by any means, but ignorant of the law. The health visitor is usually the only person who knows where they are, and will often have the confidence of the women and persuade them to become registered, but it is a most important part of the health visitor's role to maintain her relationship even with an unregistered minder in order to continue health surveillance of the children involved.

references

1. Illinworth, R. S. (1970). *The Development of the Young Child: Normal and Abnormal.* (Edinburgh: Livingstone)
2. Gesell, A. and Armatruda, C. S. (1948). *Developmental Diagnosis.* (New York: Hoeber)
3. Robson, P. (1970). Shuffling, hitching, scooting or sliding: some observations in 30 otherwise normal children. *Devel. Med. Child Neurol.*, **12**, 608
4. Harris, G. R. (1975). *The Development of Children who Shuffle.* (Institute of Child Health: University of Birmingham)
5. Thomas, A., Chess, S. and Birch, H. G. (1968). *Temperament and Behaviour Disorders in Children.* (New York: Viking Press)
6. Wood, M. E. (1973). *Children: the Development of Personality and Behaviour.* (London: Harrap)
7. Winnicott, D. W. (1957). *The Child and the Outside World.* (London: Tavistock Publications Ltd.)
8. Bell, A. Doyne (1958). The force of habit in childhood. *Lancet*, **2**, 1025
9. Reports on Health and Social Subjects. *A Nutrition Survey of Preschool Children, 1967–68.* (London: HMSO)
10. Apley, J. and MacKeith, R. C. (1962). *The Child and his Symptoms.* (Oxford: Blackwell)
11. McNeal, J. and Rogers, M. (1971). *The Multiracial School.* (London: Penguin Books)
12. Armitstead, M. (1974). *A Survey of Child Development in Caravan Dwellers.* (Institute of Child Health: University of Birmingham)
13. Karlin, I., David, K. and Guren, L. (1977). *Development and Disorders in Childhood.* (Springfield Illinois: Thomas)
14. *Handicapped Children and their Families* (1964). (Dumfermline: Carnegie United Kingdom Trust)
15. Luria, A. A. (1973). *The Working Brain.* (Harmondsworth: Penguin Books)
16. Critchley, M. (1953). *The Parietal Lobes.* (New York: Arnold)
17. Mountcastle, V. B. (1978). Brain mechanisms for directed attention. *J. R. Soc. Med.*, **71**, 14
18. Luria, A. A. (1961). *The Role of Speech in the Regulation of Normal and Abnormal Behaviour.* (New York: Liversight)
19. White, F. A. (1976). *Widening Horizons of Child Health.* (Lancaster: MTP Press)

20. Morley, M. E. (1972) *The Development and Disorders of Speech in Childhood.* (Edinburgh: Churchill Livingstone)
21. Sheridan, M. (1973). Children of 7-years with marked speech defects. *Br. J. Disord. Commun.*, **8**, 9
22. Stott, D. H. (1963). *The Social Adjustment of Children: Manual to the Bristol Social Adjustment Guide.* (London: University of London Press)
23. Rutter, M. and Martin, J. A. M. (1972). *The Child with Delayed Speech.* (London: Heinemann)
24. Ingram, T. T. S. (1972). The classification of speech and language disorders in young children. In Rutter, M. and Martin, J. A. M. (eds.) *The Child with Delayed Speech.* (London: Heinemann)
25. Wing, L. (1969). The handicaps of autistic children – a comparative study. *J. Child Psychol. Psychiatry*, **10**, 1
26. Shasby, D.M. *et al.* (1977). Epidemic measles in a highly vaccinated population. *N. Engl. J. Med.*, **296**, 585
27. Editorial (1977). Acceptance of measles vaccine. *Lancet*, **2**, 387
28. 4th report of the Medical Research Council Measles subcommittee. (1977). Clinical trial of live measles vaccine given alone and live vaccine preceded by killed vaccine. *Lancet*, **2**, 571
29. DHSS (1977). *Health And Social Services Review, 1976.* (London: HMSO)
30. Krugman, S. J. (1977). Present status of measles and rubella immunisation in the United States: a medical progress report. *J. Paediatr.*, **90**, 1
31. Miller, D. L. (1964). Frequency of complications of measles. *Br. Med. J.*, **2**, 75
32. Morley, D., Woodland, M., and Martin, W. J. (1963). Measles in Nigerian children. A study of the disease in West Africa and its manifestations in England and other countries during different epochs. *J. Hyg.*, **61**, 115
33. Dossetor, J., Whittle, H. C. and Greenwood, B. M. (1976). Persistent measles infection in malnourished children. *Br. Med. J.*, **1**, 1633
34. Buynak, E., Weibel, R., Mclean, A. and Hilleman, M. (1976). Long-term persistence of anti-body following Enders' original and More attenuated live measles virus vaccine. *Proc. Soc. Exp. Biol. Med.*, **153**, 441
35. Immunisation Programmes for Children. Report on a working group with the participation of the International Children's Centre. (Copenhagen: WHO) 1977.
36. Report of the Committee on the Child Health Services (1976). *Fit for the Future.* (London: HMSO)
37. OPCS Social Survey Division (1975). *Children's Dental Health in England and Wales, 1973.* (London: HMSO)
38. Hodges, C. H. (1974) Fluorides in paediatrics. *Am. J. Dis. Child.*, **128**, 291

39. DHSS Report no. 122 (1965). *The Fluoridation Studies in the United Kingdom and the Results Achieved after 11 years.* (London: HMSO)
40. Kennedy, D. P. (1970). School dental nurses in New Zealand. *N. Z. Med. J.*, **72**, 301
41. Mitchell, R. G. (1973). Accidents, burns and poisoning in childhood. In Forfar, J. O. and Arreil, G. C. *Textbook of Paediatrics* (Edinburgh: Churchill Livingstone)
42. European Conference of Ministers of Transport (1972). *Report of Recent Trends in Road Traffic Accidents.* (Paris: HMSO)
43. Saddler, J. (1972). Children and road safety: a survey amongst mothers. (London: HMSO)
44. Haggerty, R. J. (1959). Home accidents in childhood. *N. Engl. J. Med.*, **260**, 1322
45. MacCarthy, M. A. (1967). Selected types of poisoning as causes of accidental death. *Publ. Health Rep. Washington*, **82**, 1025
46. Editorial (1977). Emetics for acute poisoning – treatment or hazard? *Br. Med. J.*, **2**, 977
47. De Genaro, F. and Nyhan, W. L. (1971). Salt – a dangerous antidote. *J. Paediatr.*, **78**, 1048
48. Editorial (1977). Immersion and drowning in children. *Br. Med. J.*, **2**, 146
49. Keatinge, W. R. (1969). *Survival in Cold Water.* (Oxford: Blackwell)
50. Adelstein, A. M. (1977). National statistics. In Barltrop, D. (ed.) *Paediatrics and the Environment.* (London: Fellowship of Postgraduate Medicine)
51. Editorial (1976). Children who die through social disadvantage. *Br. Med. J.*, **2**, 962
52. Erikson, E. H. (1965). *Childhood and Society.* (London: Penguin Books)
53. Pitt, B. (1968). Atypical depression following childbirth. *Br. J. Psychiatry*, **114**, 1325
54. Paffenburger, R. S. (1964). Epidemiological aspects of postpartum mental illness. *Br. J. Prev. Soc. Med.*, **18**, 189
55. Brown, G. W. Bhrolchain, M. N. and Harris, T. (1975). Social class and psychiatric disturbance among women in an urban population. *Sociology*, **17**, 75
56. Richman, N. (1976). Depression in mothers of pre-school children. *J. Child Psychol. Psychiatry*, **17**, 75
57. Wolff, S. (1961). Social and family background of pre-school children with behaviour disorder attending a Child Guidance Clinic. *J. Child Psychol. Psychiatry*, **2**, 260
58. Rutter, M. (1966). *Children of Sick Parents: Maudsley Monogram.* (London: Oxford University Press)
59. Minde, K. (1976). Child psychiatry in developing countries. *J. Child Psychol. Psychiatry*, **17**, 79
60. Rutter, M. (1967). A children's behaviour questionnaire for com-

pletion by teachers. *J. Child Psychol. Psychiatry*, **8**, 1
61. Mostow, E. and Newberry, P. (1975). Work role and depression in women. *Am. J. Orthopsychiatry*, **45**, 53
62. Brown, G. W., Harris, T. O. and Peto, S. (1973). Life events and psychiatric disorders. *J. Psychol. Med.*, **3**, 159
63. Lucas, J. and McKennal, V. (1974). *The Penguin Book of Playgroups.* (London: Penguin Books)
64. The Nurseries and Childminders Act. (1948). (London: HMSO)

chapter four

the years from 3 to 5

normal development

On examination, we should see a slim child able to help dress and undress and speaking in simple sentences. By the time children begin to stand and walk, the extensor muscles of the back, neck and hips are well developed and the spine is straight. In the upright posture, the force of gravity exerted in a vertical direction causes an exaggerated lumbar lordosis and a protuberant abdomen, with an apparent knock-knee and valgus deformity of the ankles simulating flat feet[1]. To measure the degree of knock-knee, the child should be facing straight forward, with the feet straight and the medial surface of the knees just touching, not overlapping, and the distance between the medial malleoli of the ankles measured. A survey of 1000 children[2] found four grades of knock-knee. Grade 1 was less than 2.5 cm and found in 26% of the children studied; Grade 2 was 2.5 to 5.0 cm, the most common measurement and found in 52% of the children studied; Grade 3 was 5.0 to 7.5 cm and found in 22% of the children studied; Grade 4 was 7.5 cm or greater and found in 2% of the children studied. There were no sex differences. The children with knock-knee were heavier.

As with the mild to moderate degree of bowing of the legs that occurs in infancy, mild to moderate knock-knee corrects spontaneously with growth and development[1]. No treatment is indicated except to reassure the parents, unless the degree of knock-knee is very severe or secondary to some other disorder such as rickets or obesity. True flatfoot is very rare although an apparent flatfoot in young children is relatively common. To assess the feet of children they should be asked to stand on their toes or sit on a chair with their feet off the ground, when the true arch of the foot can be seen.

motor

Motor development ranges from the 3-year-old who will be able to go upstairs alone one foot on each step but may come down backwards or only if helped, to competent descent by 4½–5 years. Where children live in bungalows or flats, enquiry about the child's ability to climb and jump or to get in and out of cars and buses will give a reasonable estimate of gross motor development.

Co-ordination and fine motor development are best tested at the time of examination by finger–thumb apposition and rapid tapping and by observing the child's ability to draw, build with bricks, handle screw toys, do up and undo buttons and laces and to find and pick up small objects on the floor[3]. Small children delight in helping the clumsy doctor so that judicious dropping of objects can be employed to test the child. Sequential finger to thumb apposition and rapid tapping with each hand separately may be too difficult for some 3–4-year-olds and clapping hands may be used as an alternative.

Manipulation of toys, putting bricks together to form a train of 3–4 bricks or a tower of 8 bricks when shown, explores the child's improving eye–hand co-ordination. Manipulation of pencils in drawing first a straight line at 2+ years, then a circle at 3 years, is evidence of the ability to concentrate and increasing motor control and visual perception. As children get older, their representation of the human figure in the Goodenough Draw a Man Test (see page 147) may act as a guide to their ability and a monitor of the parents' assurance that their children are allowed to use pencils and crayons at home. In many poor families, children may not have experienced the use of pencils and paints at home. The cost of paper and colouring books is out of the reach of some poorer families though many of them buy a daily paper or can buy scraps of cheap wall paper. Both newspaper and scrap paper can be used as an alternative and very effective resource for drawing or colouring with water colours, crayons or pencils for young children.

Preference of hand, foot, eye and ear is usually established by the second birthday[4]. The child reported to have an established hand preference since infancy is likely to have a hemiplegia. Preference is not dominance although these are intertwined. Why test for preference? Firstly, to protect the natural left-hander. Some parents regard left-handedness as abnormal and attempt to make their left-handed child use the right hand. Parents who are right-handed may find their left-handed child clumsy or slow when there is difficulty in teaching the child how to do up buttons or tie knots. Advising the mother that the way to do this is to sit behind her child with both of them facing a mirror so that the left-handed child gets the correct image may relieve tension at home and the guilt of the child and the mother. It is usual for the mother to take a large share of the blame, where this is apportioned by families, as well as the burden if a child is thought to be slow or handicapped.

Secondly, it is often thought that mixed preference may be a sign of continuing clumsiness or future problems in reading and writing but this is not always so[5]. Children with mixed hand–eye co-ordination and some natural left-handers do appear to use inversions and reversions of letters such as *p* and *b*, *g* and *d*, until they are older, up to 8, 9 or 10 years, and more often than children with a pure right preference or dominance. To mention this to parents and teachers and reassure them that it is normal helps to alleviate anxiety. Educationalists in some areas have introduced programmes in schools to encourage preference for right or left in children when preference is mixed, to improve the child's ability in literacy and numeracy and to overcome clumsiness. Whether this programme works or whether it is the interest and encouragement given to the individual child by the teacher which is effective, is not known. Over-enthusiasm on the part of educational advisers for these methods needs to be tempered especially in the case of the child with a handicap. One such adviser had thought that a partially sighted child should be encouraged to develop right eye as well as hand preference although his left eye was his better one for vision. This possibly disastrous course of action was prevented by the concern of his teachers and parents in requesting urgent medical support to veto the action.

When testing for preference, it is essential not to clue the child. One must never offer the object to be picked up to one hand or the other and both the child's hands must be free. This can be combined with testing for foot preference when the child after kicking a brick is asked to pick the brick up. A ball should not be used for kicking as it is thought that children see so many footballers on television kicking with their right foot that they imitate this action rather than using their preferred foot. This supports the view that preference may be socially conditioned[6]. For eye preference, a sheet of plain paper with a small hole in the centre (if the hole is too big, children will put it on the bridge of their nose) or a roll of paper (although small children tend to squash the latter) is effective. For the preferred ear, a watch with a quiet tick is placed on the table and the child asked if he or she can hear the tick – children will either pick the watch up to listen or, if the table is low enough, incline their ear to the watch on the table.

social

Children now begin to understand the similarities and differences between themselves and other people in relation to age, sex and social roles and will act this out in play[7]. Their view is still egocentric and they regard themselves as the cause of any action which appears to distress them or the adults around them[8], such as Andrew, aged 4 years, whose mother had been recommended for a home delivery for her second baby. Her husband arrived home from work and was preparing an evening meal when she went into rapid labour. Immediate concern for his wife led the father to get the midwife and the family doctor. Four hours later, with new baby safely delivered, the father realized that Andrew had not been seen for some time. Andrew was eventually found in the garage crying whilst trying to paint himself all over, hair included, with blue paint – a very apt colour scheme.

Children first learn to understand actions and much later expressions, that is they will understand the significance of laughter or tears before understanding a happy or sad expression[9]. Similarly, the gravity of any act is judged by the amount of damage done not by the intention behind the act, e.g. it is more serious to break a big vase while helping mummy than to break a small one while stealing food from the larder.

play

Children play with pleasure and play has an important role in social and emotional development[10]. Play helps children to release aggression in a socially acceptable manner. Young aggressive adolescents, sent by their schools to help the staff at playgroups and nurseries and to learn about the care and needs of young children, find the atmosphere of the playgroup or nursery therapeutic. The adolescents enjoy the play as much as the children. Teachers report these young people to be more relaxed and improved in behaviour during these episodes. Play helps children to cope with anxiety and to gain experience of life.

All children use play to relieve their anxieties and to act out their fantasies[10]. A child who is able to play, either alone or with other children, has a natural outlet which will enable the child to develop normally despite other stresses. Children under five can be seen apparently playing together but this is not usual until the child has ceased to speak egocentrically. Children are unable to combine effectively together in an activity until they can speak to each other in a meaningful way[10]. Three-year-olds cannot attend to more than one person at a time and need to be in small groups.

All children play fathers and mothers, often acting out the adult sexual roles in relationship to each other. Children's play is enriched with sexual symbols and ideas and will involve physical excitement which needs to be relieved by achieving a climax such as a capture, prize or special treat. If the excitement is not relieved before the child is put to bed, night terrors may occur, disturbing the child's sleep. Then the mother or father is needed immediately to reassure the child[10].

Imaginary companions are a normal phenomenon, which occurs most commonly in children of 3–4 years of age, and most frequently in only children[11]. Research on gifted children[12] showed that 85% of the girls and 51% of the boys had imaginary playmates. Piaget[13] considered this type of play was used by the child as a means of expressing and extending reality. Symbolic and fantasy play allows the child to relive and cope with experiences which might otherwise be too painful or threatening. Imaginary companions also appear in neurotic and maladjusted children, probably associated with the child's distortion of reality and to satisfy longings frustrated by reality.

Masturbation, when it occurs, is healthy and normal unless it is compulsive and excessive[10]. Masturbation which is compulsive, like head-banging, rocking or excessive tics, is evidence of an excessive anxiety and it is the underlying anxiety that should be dealt with, not the masturbation. Excessive masturbation of an exhausting nature may happen with the seriously mentally ill child or the severely mentally handicapped child and the masturbation must be repressed. Any child with a behaviour disorder that is excessive and persistent to the point of embarrassment should be referred to a child psychiatrist.

vision testing

Testing vision and hearing in 3–5-year-olds is a more co-operative procedure. Single letter cards, used in vision testing at 6 metres (20 feet), may give misleading results and need to be used with care, but give useful practice to children in matching shapes and letters. Letter cards such as the Snellen Chart should be used for testing vision as soon as possible[14]. The latter can be used before a child has learnt to read all the letters and still give correct results – a 5-year-old whose mother was worried about her vision and who had had three tests with the single letter eye card had her visual acuity each time reported as 6/6. The child could read sufficient letters to use a Snellen Chart and her vision tested by this method was found to be 6/18. It appears, despite refractive errors, easier to recognize a single letter alone yet, when the same letter is in a line with others, some form of telescopic fusion takes place which shows up the defect in visual acuity. Near vision can be tested with specialist cards of print or letters and is as important as testing distant vision in assessing vision handicap – if near vision is reduced and not improved by glasses, the child will probably need additional visual aids at school or special education in a school for partially sighted children.

'Hundreds and Thousands' sugar cake decorations may be used to screen near vision with the unintelligent or overactive child. David, the only child of a young, single mother, suffered a series of unsatisfactory child minders before admission to a day care centre at 3½ years of age. He was a well grown little boy, socially competent at table and toilet. His speech and language were at an 18/12 level being mostly single words with dyslalia and echolalia. His attention span was about 60 seconds. There appeared to be no squint, although he had not been seen by the orthoptist in infancy. He was unable to co-operate for vision and hearing screening although in play and socially these appeared normal.

David was conditioned for his vision screening test by attending when the new children admitted to the centre came for their tests. In the meantime he was seen by the specialist team for hearing testing and a speech therapist. Hearing was normal and the speech therapist reported that his speech, though intelligible, was bizarre due to irrelevant responses and echolalia. Concentration was poor. A programme of language development was advised for the staff at the centre and David was reviewed after six months. Within a few weeks, David was able to co-operate with a test of visual acuity and failed his near vision test ('Hundreds and Thousands') although his distant vision was normal. He was seen at the specialist clinic, hypermetropia confirmed and glasses prescribed.

Five months later he was reviewed by the speech therapist whose report is reproduced:

> 'David has shown remarkable improvement as regards his speech and language development although apparently his behaviour is still erratic. On the previous occasion 7/12 ago he could not deal with assessment material but his vision had not then been corrected. This, and a good stimulating environment, has obviously transformed him and I doubt if he will need speech therapy if progress continues.'

The caring, stimulating environment and the correction of his sensory deprivation by the provision of glasses has enabled David to make up for some of his early deprivation. Labelling such a child as 'slow' or 'mentally handicapped', instead of conditioning him to co-operate with tests of vision and hearing, is a failure of the health services for young children. Examination of children must be carried out by people with knowledge and experience.

It will be noted that David's behaviour is still described as erratic and may deteriorate in the wider setting of the infant class where there is one adult to 20–30 children. In the infant school David will be part of a larger social group of the school (100+), whereas in his day care centre there is one adult to 7–10 children in a setting of 30–40 people.

If the local infant schools accept rising fives, it may be thought that such a child as David, in the euphoria of his rapid progress, is ready to start school early, often the wish of delighted parents and care staff. However, a prolonged stay in a stable environment is essential to allow children like David to consolidate their gains and develop confidence in their own ability. This is a fine decision and depends on local circumstances and the facilities available, the important point being not to disturb the improving influence until the child is ready. The help of a psychologist in difficult cases is essential.

Another important consideration to be resolved for David's future development is the result of his mother being a single parent working long hours. Hence, there will be the additional problem of care after school and in the school holidays. Many day care centres and nurseries will help initially in taking their own children after school but there is a limit to the number of children and for how long centres for pre-school children can cope with the larger, older schoolchild. It is not good for the older schoolchild either. Once he starts a school day, does David become a latch-key child or again the victim of a procession of unsatisfactory minders? It might be that, even in one so young, weekly boarding will have to be considered.

hearing testing (see also appendix 1)

Hearing should be carefully screened to exclude the insidious onset of conductive loss due to recurrent middle ear infection and glue ear. New cases of sensori-neural loss may occur where disease or disorder of the central nervous system causes a lesion of the auditory nerve and central auditory connections, such as following meningitis, whether bacterial or viral, cerebral tumour, and head injury, or damage to the inner ear, especially the cochlea, following the use of ototoxic drugs such as streptomycin, neomycin and kanamycin. Children with secondary hearing loss will have had some period of normal hearing and are particularly difficult to recognize without skilled testing, especially when the hearing loss is unilateral[15].

Conductive hearing loss may be intermittent. Intermittent loss may have profound effects on a child's language development and create serious problems in school. Recurrent otitis media is not always accompanied by pain or the child may not complain of pain, which makes examination of eardrums a necessary part of hearing screening. It is wise to exclude dental disease when earache is associated with a normal eardrum.

A conductive hearing loss must be excluded when a child has had a recurrent upper respiratory tract infection (URTI) and where parents complain that a child is 'lazy' or 'doesn't pay attention unless they shout'. Pure tone audiometry or impedance testing is recommended on more than one occasion. An interval of six weeks between tests is suggested[16]. Children with minor hearing deficits show considerable educational retardation as a group, with restricted language development due to impaired auditory processing skills[17]. This group of children are also prone to emotional disorders, as many as 30% needing referral to child guidance clinics[18].

Careful scrutiny of a child's response to high frequency sounds, and of the development of the use of sentences, will screen some of the sensori-neural high frequency losses. Failure in the development of speech and language is sometimes assigned incorrectly to the home background. A 3-year-old was admitted to hospital with a febrile convulsion and was noted to have speech delay. A hearing test was not done although a place was obtained for the child in a day nursery to stimulate his speech development. His high tone hearing loss was not diagnosed until routine screening at school, and was sufficiently severe to require admission to a school for partially-hearing children.

speech and language

Between 2 and 6 years of age a child's vocabulary increases tenfold, and, between 3 and 4 years of age, a child's speech becomes grammatically more correct[19]. A child's articulation should enable him to be understood by the adult with whom he is speaking. Parents can become used to their child's abnormal speech pattern and, where doubt exists, one should ask about the intelligibility of the child's speech outside the immediate family circle – does a member of the family always interpret? When asking a child his name, it is worthwhile finding out from the parents beforehand the name used for the child at home. This may be the second given name or a diminutive or, with people of other languages, a diminutive in their own tongue. If these precautions are not taken, the examiner may not understand what a small child with infantile articulation is saying, and the evident lack of comprehension will lose that child's co-operation.

A child's co-operation in a speech and language assessment may be difficult to obtain. Comprehension and inner language may be observed at play and tested with small toys by pretending to put them away and asking for each toy separately. The correctly given toys are put in the box and the incorrectly given toys ignored. Prepositions can be tested by asking the child to put one toy beside another – the dog beside the car, the doll on the chair. Speech disorders and serious delay in development of expressive speech should be referred to the otologist for assessment of hearing and to the speech therapist for assessment of speech and language. Delay and abnormality are never due to laziness or tongue tie and will not get better 'in time' or when the child starts school.

It is sometimes necessary to take court action where a child is deprived of treatment by his parents. Mary, a 4-year-old with an extensive cleft palate, was referred for special education as her parents had failed all hospital follow-up appointments with both the paediatrician and the surgeon since the primary lip repair when Mary was 8/12 of age. A clinic appointment with the senior clinical medical officer and the speech therapist was not kept despite promises by the mother to the health visitor and family doctor. A morning home visit by the senior medical officer, without warning, found the family at home.

Mary appeared to be an intelligent child with retarded language and expressive speech development, the latter being completely unintelligible. She appeared to understand what was said to her. There was an extensive palatal cleft but not wide separation. Her eardrums were normal. When pressed, her mother denied any difficulty in understanding Mary's speech. The interview and examination were undertaken in the family living room, where the television was blaring forth for the benefit of the mother's profoundly deaf father who lived with the family.

The parents were advised on the importance of treatment and the serious problems Mary would face at school if treatment were not undertaken. The mother agreed to keep an appointment at the hospital to see the surgeon so that the palate repair could be arranged. At the same time Mary would see the speech therapist and would have her hearing tested. The parents were gently reminded that it was against the law[20] in England and Wales for parents to deny their children necessary treatment to ensure normal development and failure on their part could mean court action.

The initial appointment was not kept and proceedings for a care order were put into effect. If the magistrate agreed with the request for a care order, Mary would live at home but the Director of the Social Services Department, having parental rights, would be able to ensure the child's attendance at outpatients, her admission to hospital and give permission for surgical treatment if that were necessary. No actual proceedings in this case had to be undertaken as Mary's parents agreed to her hospital treatment and speech therapy. Surgery was completed and, although Mary has failed her most recent appointments for therapy, she is now attending school regularly and can continue her therapy at the school clinic.

Young children may be fluent in using language but the meaning of the words used will be quite different to the adult concept, e.g. 'Jenny is easy to see', for the under fives, means that Jenny is doing the seeing[21]. The four-year-old may understand morning and afternoon but will not know the days of the week or be able to tell the time until 5–7 years of age and it is the understanding of time that allows us to develop our concepts of the future.

In learning language from the adults around them, children are sharply divided by their social background: all parents use a 'restricted' code, such as 'shut the door' which is rigid, predictable and thinks only in the present, whereas children from good linguistic backgrounds are also exposed to a more 'elaborate' code, such as 'please close the door quietly dear as mummy has a headache' which conveys shades of meaning, is more subtle, has a wider range and allows feelings to be expressed. In child rearing, the 'elaborate' code is thought to lead to greater inner restraint and control, whereas the 'restricted' code relies on strength and dominance to control behaviour[22].

preventive medicine

immunization

Pertussis vaccine should not be given after 3 years of age. Between 4 and 5 years of age, booster doses of diphtheria and tetanus toxoid with oral polio vaccine should be given to all children to maintain immunity[23]. Young children in day nurseries and nursery schools are at greater risk of contact with infection. Prevention of tetanus by active immunization is of prime importance. Since 1966 it has been realized that tetanus toxoid may cause an adverse reaction[24], usually not serious but to be avoided. Frequent booster doses of tetanus toxoid are no longer necessary as adsorbed toxoid, introduced into the United Kingdom in 1963, gives a more durable immunity than was previously recognized[25]. Following the booster dose at 5 years of age, ten-year intervals for further boosters are recommended[25]. If primary immunization was not completed, and, as less than five years will have elapsed since the single injection, two further injections six to twelve months apart should be given.

accidents

Starting school means more independence for the child and greater involvement with traffic with a rapidly rising incidence of accidents outside the home.

The commonest cause of admission to hospital for children under 5 years of age is the accidental ingestion of drugs[26]. The commonest cause of accidental death in this age group is the ingestion of tricyclic antidepressants[27]. The use of childproof containers is one aspect of prevention, the other aspect being care on the part of the doctor in prescribing dangerous medicines for any member of a family when there are young children in the household.

where should I go?

Day nurseries, playgroups and day care are an acceptable form of pre-school care for children before they enter school at the compulsory school age of 5 years. Parents have increasingly requested that more nursery school provision be made available for all children between 3 and 5 years. Nursery education may be made available in either nursery schools or nursery classes: both are a part of primary education. The nursery school will have its own head teacher and staff, whereas the nursery class will be an integral part of the local infant or primary school with a single head teacher. It is normal school health practice for the school nurse to visit the nursery departments – schools or classes – weekly, as the incidence of infection and developmental problems is higher in this age group.

Nursery education is rapidly becoming more common but at present there are insufficient schools for the demand. Many schools allow half-day attendance and make it possible for a larger group of children to attend. This may lead to additional strains on the staff and an additional hazard when infections occur. The important part of nursery education is size of school and of class. Small children cannot relate to more than one adult at a time and may be overwhelmed by the school environment. Some children may be very shy or aggressive before they settle down. For a few children, a long period of separation from their mothers is unwise, especially for a whole school day, and, if insisted upon, will cause severe distress to the child. Nursery school staff are aware of the problem of distress, and, if this is present, encourage the mother to keep her child at home for a further period of time; it will be necessary to ensure that this enlightened attitude continues when there is no shortage of nursery school places.

Most children undoubtedly derive considerable benefit from a nursery education in social and cognitive development, especially children from the less stimulating home. Nursery education for the handicapped child is of a more specialized kind, as are special schools, and, as has already been mentioned, this type of education may be made possible from a very young age, even below 3 years. Special school nursery departments are always attached to a parent school and will fall into the definition of nursery classes. Special schools' nursery departments have the specialized educational facilities of the parent school and access to the special resources of the School Health Service and the Hospital Paediatric Services.

references

1. Tachdijan. M. O. (1972). *Paediatric Orthopaedics.* (Philadelphia: W. B. Saunders & Co.)
2. Morley, A. J. M. (1957). Knock knee in children. *Br. Med. J.*, **2**, 976
3. Paine, R. S. and Oppé, T. E. (1966). *Neurological Examination of Children.* (London: Spastics Society and Heinemann)
4. Griffiths, R. (1954). *The Abilities of Babies.* (London: University of London Press)
5. Douglas, J. W. B., Ross, J. M. and Cooper, J. E. (1967). The relationship between handedness, attainment and adjustment in a national sample of schoolchildren. *Educ. Res.*, **9**, 223
6. Ausubel, D. P. (1958). *Theory and Problems of Child Development.* (New York: Grune & Stratton)
7. Wood, M. E. (1973). *Children: the Development of Personality and Behaviour.* (London: Harrap)
8. Piaget, J. (1929). *The Child's Conception of the World.* (New York: Harcourt Brace Jovanovich)
9. Honkavarra, S. (1961). The psychology of expression. *Br. J. Psychol.* 32
10. Winnicott, D. W. (1957). *The Child and the Outside World.* (London: Tavistock Publications Ltd.)
11. Valentine, C. W. (1970). *The Normal Child and some of his Abnormalities.* (Harmondsworth: Penguin Books)
12. Terman, L. M. (1926). *Genetic Studies of Genius.* (Stanford: Stanford University Press)
13. Piaget, J. (1951). *Play, Dreams and Imitation in Childhood.* (New York: Norton)
14. Wybar, K. (1974). *Ophthalmology.* (London: Baillière Tindall)
15. Peckham, C. S., Sheridan, M. and Butler, N. R. (1972). School attainment of seven-year-old children with hearing difficulties. *Devel. Med. Child Neurol.*, **5**, 592
16. Brooks, D. N. (1977). Auditory screening – time for re-appraisal. *Public Health*, **91**, 282

17. Lewis, N. (1976). Otitis media and linguistic incompetence. *Arch. Otolaryngol.*, **102**, 87
18. Meadow, K. P. and Schlesinger, H. S. (1971). The prevalence of behaviour problems in a population of deaf schoolchildren. *Am. Ann. Deaf*, **3**, 346
19. Smith, M. E. (1926). An investigation of the sentence and the extent of vocabulary in young children. Studies in Child Welfare, University of Iowa
20. Children and Young Persons Act. (1970). (London: HMSO)
21. Cromer, R. F. (1970). Children are nice to understand. *Br. J. Psychol.*, 61
22. Bernstein, B. (1961). Social class and linguistic development. In Halsey, A. H., Floud, J. and Anderson, C. A. (eds). *Education, Economy and Society* (New York: The Free Press)
23. DHSS (1978). *Revised Schedule on Vaccination and Immunisation Procedures*, (London: HMSO)
24. White, W. G. *et al* (1969). Duration of immunity after active immunisation against tetanus. *Lancet*, **2**, 95
25. Trinca, J. C. (1965). Active immunisation against tetanus: the need for a single purpose toxoid. *Med. J. Aust.*, **2**, 116
26. Medicines Commission (1974). *Report on the Presentation of Medicine in relation to Child Safety*. (London: HMSO)
27. OPCS (1978). *Deaths by Accidental Poisoning 1962–76*. (London: HMSO)

chapter five

the years from 5 to 7

the primary school

Parents are responsible for ensuring that their children receive efficient full time education by 'regular attendance at school or otherwise'[1]. The majority of children are ready to start school and to be part of a larger group at 5 years of age, although some anxiety and stress is inevitable in leaving home and mother. At school, children become involved in making new friends and learning in a structured environment. Children who have previously attended a nursery school are at an initial advantage in having experienced school life[2].

Children deprived socially and linguistically are likely to find entry to school extremely difficult. For these children, where attitudes at home are to the present and not to the future, attitudes at school to work and learning for the future are alien[3]. In such a deprived group of children, conscious control of emotion and behaviour is often not established, as reliance at home is placed on the greater physical strength of the adult.

Other children who may have difficulty when starting school are those who are overprotected and who are only children, especially boys[4]. These children and their mothers need support to encourage attendance. The mother with an immature personality may show jealousy of the affection her child has for the teacher, not recognizing that there is no competition, and will endeavour to keep the child away from school on the slightest pretext. This type of situation, where the child becomes a failure due to lack of attendance, may be a precursor to truancy.

Between 5 and 7 years, co-operative play is more common especially with children who know each other, although play is often dominated by one child and the other children given roles to perform. Children are becoming aware of rules in games and enjoy rules as this gives them a sense of security[3]. They still need the help of their parents in play and their parents' interest and concern for the problems and joys of their wider world at school.

Knowledge and understanding of the motives of people is limited in the under sevens and, when making judgements, they are more likely to look at the consequences of an action rather than the reasons behind it. Children's likes and dislikes of adults and other children will centre around the appearance and the environment of those persons rather than the feelings and the sentiments expressed by them[5].

Many mothers will arrange to start work when their youngest child starts school, forgetting that a whole day away from their mother is too long for some small children, as this will involve staying at school for the midday meal. If excessive anxiety is being shown by the child such as nightmares, behaviour changes, recurrent vomiting or abdominal pain with no physical cause, the school doctor will advise the mother and the teacher about management. In some cases of anxiety it may suffice to allow the child to come home for the midday meal. In more severe cases, with the co-operation of the school and the Education Authority, the child may be allowed to attend for half-days only. This may be necessary for as short a time as a week or at the most for 5 weeks, i.e. half a school term. If the symptoms expressed by the child do not show signs of resolving within that time, the more expert help of the Child Guidance Clinic is needed (see chapter 8).

Children with moderate handicap may respond and benefit from education in the infant department of their local school. One such boy, an only child, was referred for nursery school with a behaviour problem at home. He had developed a neurotic illness following admission to hospital for investigation of dwarfism. The paediatrician and child psychiatrist felt that this boy was suffering from dwarfism due to deprivation. His intelligence was within the normal range and his play was normal. There was no evidence of excessive fantasy but his speech and language development were retarded. His parents had separated during his mother's pregnancy, although at 4 years of age, when admitted to school, his mother had a stable relationship with a man accepted by the child as 'Dad'. He was admitted to the nursery class attached to the infant school and was noted by the teaching staff to be remarkably small and singularly capable of getting into trouble. At seven years of age, he is working at a good average level, his educational attainments are average and his language development is normal. He still finds it difficult to curb his impetuosity and he is still below the 2nd centile in height although his growth is following the normal curve. At home, his mother and her cohabitee have married and the family relationship appears settled.

Class sizes should be small and teaching so structured that all the children in the class will benefit. Socially, many handicapped children will mature in such an environment and attending a local school will mean less travelling, a shorter, less tiring day for the young handicapped child and the possibility of more independence as he gets older.

If it is policy to encourage the integration of handicapped pupils in to ordinary schools, as it has been in some education authorities for many years, reinforced by the Report of the

Warnock Committee[6], certain criteria must be met. Class size, teaching ability and interest are of first importance. Professional advice on the nature of the handicap and how it affects the child must be made available to the class teacher, with the support of specialist teachers and advice from the school doctor, the school nurse and the school psychologist. Additional non-teaching help may be needed for toileting, washing and feeding. Medical advice and support and daily nurse attendance should be made available for the staff at schools where there are children on continuous medication which has to be given at school. Even with all these precautions, the decision to integrate the handicapped child may be wrong, and it is imperative that, whatever judgements are made, they are for the happiness, benefit and the ultimate educational attainment of the child and not because they make the parents, the professionals or the members of the school staff and the education authority feel a glow of self-satisfaction, which is easily interpreted as being in the best interests of the child.

The medical examination of children at school has rightly been criticized[7], both on the time made available for the examination of the children and the premises used. The education authorities have a duty to make suitable premises available and most schools will endeavour to provide rooms with privacy and sufficient space. If facilities are inadequate the children should be examined at the local clinic or health centre. The amount of time given to each child will depend on the age of the children to be seen, the problems elicited or referred, other facilities available and the family's social situation. The importance of pre-school and school medical examinations is to allow the parents' concern about their children to be aired. If the examination is only satisfying the doctor about the physical health of the child, it is virtually useless.

medical problems

Problems that particularly worry teachers in the infant's school are those of the aggressive, thieving, anxious, withdrawn or attention-seeking child[8]. These are the children that the school doctor will be asked to see. The clinical medical officer plays a major role in the management of the simple psychological problems both of the pre-school and the school child. This may account for the low proportion of such problems: 3.5% in over a thousand children who were attending their family doctors for treatment[9].

incontinence

Other conditions occurring in the schoolchild which are referred to the school doctor are incontinence of urine or faeces or both. Failure to become continent by the time a child starts school may be very distressing for the child and parents and is always so if there is daytime incontinence. Many schools can cope with a variety of problems but the smell and unpleasantness associated with incontinence during the day may be too much for the teacher and the other children.

Most children will become continent for bowel and bladder by day and night between 3 and 5 years. After this age, nocturnal enuresis is said to decline by 20% per year as children mature and become more competent[10]. When a child who has been dry becomes enuretic under the stress of change, such as starting or changing schools, both the parents and the child should be reassured about the outcome although the wise doctor will review the situation at an early stage.

Persistent enuresis requires a detailed history of voiding, and, for boys, evidence should be obtained from the father or by direct observation as the mother may be unreliable. Any history of frequency, urgency, difficulty in starting the stream, dribbling, interruption of the stream, soiling or constipation, including details of preceding gastro-intestinal and urinary tract infection should be included. Examination will include a neurological examination and exclusion of infection and infestation in the renal and GI tracts. Screening for bacteriuria is important in the under fives. New kidney scars rarely develop and intrarenal reflux does not occur after the age of 4 years[11]. The combination of infection and vesicoureteric reflux in a child under 4 years of age will lead to renal scarring with permanent damage and eventually renal failure[12], whereas studies[13,14] in older children, aged 5 to 15 years, have shown that kidneys that were not scarred initially remained unscarred and growth was not impaired in the presence of persistent bacteriuria or reflux or both. However, in children with scarred kidneys, reduction of exposure to bacteriuria by treatment may prevent new scar formation as these only occurred in the untreated group, although treatment did not forestall the progression of established renal scars[15]. In the child under 4 years of age, urinary tract infection with reflux, especially the more severe form of reflux associated with pyelotubular backflow, needs longterm antibiotic treatment[12] to prevent chronic pyelonephritis and early development of raised blood pressure. Surgical treatment of the more severe grades of reflux may be necessary[15]. Bacteriuria in older children who are enuretic is found most commonly in girls, whether day or night time enuretics, and was thought to be the result of wet underclothing rather than the cause of the enuresis, as eradication of the infection did not alter the pattern of wetting[16].

Nocturnal enuresis is more commonly a developmental variant and not due to a physical disorder. There is not uncommonly a positive family history. Other possible causes need to be kept in mind. A mentally handicapped child will be more likely to be enuretic as a reflection of his developmental age compared with his chronological age. Epilepsy should be excluded. Seizures are more common at night and it is possible that a transitory rise in intracranial pressure, which occurs on going to sleep and waking, may give rise to a seizure and so cause bed wetting. Psychiatric disturbance, as evidenced by neuroticism in girls and antisocial behaviour in boys, was more common in day and night enuretics, associated with urgency in both sexes and soiling in boys. Children with nocturnal enuresis alone differed little from normal controls[16].

management of nocturnal enuresis

Nocturnal enuresis is defined as persistent, involuntary

micturition during sleep in the absence of demonstrable pathology[17].

Having taken the history and examined the child, the problem is discussed with the child and the parents. Simple explanation that nocturnal enuresis is not uncommon will help to relieve anxiety in the child and reassure the parents. If the parents wish to discuss the problem with the doctor alone, the child should be told what the discussion will be about and invited to return when the method of treatment has been decided. Parents are asked not to restrict drinks in the evening, there being no evidence that this is effective. Parents may continue potting the child before they themselves go to bed if they are already doing so.

The simplest form of treatment is to use a calendar on which the child is asked to colour in or to paste a star on those days when his bed is dry. Regular follow-up by interested and confident medical and nursing staff is necessary.

Where this simple form of treatment is unsuccessful and the child is happy and settled at school, the enuresis alarm is used[18]. The alarm consists of a pad which is placed under the child's bottom sheet and connected to an alarm buzzer. As soon as the child starts to urinate, the circuit is complete, the buzzer sounds and wakes the child. If the child does not wake the parents must wake him. A popular child psychiatrist has suggested that the alarm works by waking everyone in the household and the child is coerced into being continent so as not to disturb everyone.

By establishing a conditioned response a considerable success will ensue. The alarm buzzer is explained to the parents and the child and demonstrated to them. The demonstrator must not forget that the pad is urine-sensitive and will not respond to water[19]. Regular follow-up by the doctor and the nurse is essential to ensure that the child is not being conditioned to failure by faulty equipment or inadequate explanation, and a home visit may be necessary. The buzzer alarm must be used every night and continued in use for four consecutive weeks of dry beds to establish a cure. Four months is considered a fair trial[19].

Tricyclic antidepressants such as imipramine and amitriptyline may be used in older children, i.e. those over 7 years of age. These drugs are thought to have a cholinergic effect on the bladder[10] although their mode of action is uncertain. Children tend to become dry whilst taking these drugs but are said to relapse when the drugs are stopped. Therefore they are useful for short-term effect. Longterm use needs further investigation.

bowel problems

Constipation is unusual in breast-fed infants, delays up to ten days between the passage of stools being regarded as normal. Bottle-fed infants on concentrated feeds will dehydrate their stools to enable urine solute clearance to occur and, where this happens, the babies may only pass stools with considerable strain and with the risk of an anal tear causing pain and spasm and constipation. Additional water is needed to correct this situation. True constipation must always be regarded seriously and not allowed to become chronic. Chronic constipation with soiling occurs in 1.32% of children over the age of 4 years, the ratio of boys to girls[20] being 3 : 1. Constipation is defined as difficulty or delay in the passage of faeces; soiling is defined as the frequent passage of loose or semi-solid stools into clothing; encopresis is the passage of normal stools into abnormal places including clothes[21].

Many children with constipation or overflow incontinence will respond to laxatives, simple psychotherapy and attention to diet[22]. In a study[23] of 106 children who failed to respond to these simple measures, 10 children had Hirschsprung's disease and 10 children had a failure of the anal sphincter to relax in response to rectal distension (Hirschsprung-like activity). These pathological conditions are often missed due to the mistaken belief that soiling does not occur in Hirschsprung's disease. There is also a failure to recognize the miserable existence of these children, and the innumerable humiliations they have to endure, both at home and at school, as parents try desperately to train the child to be acceptable socially. The best screening procedure is ano-rectal manometry, a safe and reliable procedure[24]. Where investigation is normal and other evidence of deep emotional disturbance exists, the child should be referred to the child psychiatrist.

allergy

Other common disorders are asthma and eczema, allergic disorder being the most common disability found in a follow-up[25] of 10-year-old children with an incidence of 13.5%. Many adults regard asthma as a recurrent illness, thinking the patient to be physically fit in between attacks, whereas asthma may cause serious physical handicap and, in a very severe form, can be a killing disease[26]. Factors adversely affecting the longterm prognosis over 20 years[27] are a positive family history of atopic disease, a history or presence of infantile eczema in the patient, and the absence of breast feeding or the limitation of breast feeding to less than a week as breast milk protects the baby against infection with respiratory syncytial virus (RS virus)[28]. The age of onset does not appear to affect the longterm prognosis nor do positive skin tests although positive skin tests are associated with severity of onset[27].

Early physiotherapy and a suitable drug regimen will enable most children to attend ordinary school. Special schooling may be necessary if a child is missing time from school, and, in a few cases, residential school will produce an improvement in the affected child's health and educational ability. If it is necessary to alter a child's day at school for any reason, the change must be discussed with the head teacher before being proposed to the parents as any alteration in the school timetable for an individual child may create serious difficulty for the teaching staff.

epilepsy

It is estimated that there are 60000 schoolchildren with epilepsy in England and Wales[29]; the Isle of Wight survey found an incidence of 8.9 per 1000 children[30]. Monitoring of blood levels of anticonvulsants has led to better control of seizures with less sleepiness and personality change, allowing most children with epilepsy to be educated in ordinary schools. A small number of children, whose seizures are difficult to control or who have other handicaps, need to attend special schools. Boys rather than girls are more likely to have behavioural disturbance[31]. Petit mal makes its appearance in the early school years, and, if not recognized, will result in educational retardation and learning problems. Every child with epilepsy needs to be given the opportunity to fulfil his academic ability.

Children with epilepsy should know what tablets they are taking, and how often and why they need to take them. Compliance in drug administration can often be obtained in adolescents as they must be free of fits for three years if they wish to drive a car[32]. No child with epilepsy should be allowed to go swimming alone. Advice will be necessary for the parents and the teachers of individual children, depending on their seizures, on whether the children can ride bicycles, climb wall bars and later take part in rock and mountain climbing.

diabetes mellitus

The incidence of diabetes is reported[30] as 1.2/1000 in schoolchildren, juvenile diabetics forming 10–14% of the total diabetic population[33]. Children with diabetes must learn to be competent in measuring and administering their insulin and in recognizing the symptoms and treatment and taking precautions to prevent hypoglycaemic attacks. They should understand their diet and the need for additional food before violent exercise. Most paediatricians will undertake this type of counselling. Nevertheless, despite recommendations to the contrary, older children and adolescents[34] are admitted under the care of adult physicians, who are less likely to counsel the anxious parent in the importance of their child's independence at the right age and may delay in giving advice to the child on self-management. Although diabetic retinopathy has not been seen in children under 10 years of age, 4% of the registered blind aged 15–29 years in England and Wales owe their blindness to diabetes[35].

Better information on maintenance therapy, advice and sympathetic understanding of their fears and anxieties given to schoolchildren with chronic disorders may reduce their resistance to continued medication when adolescent and help prevent the high rate of psychiatric illness, even suicide[36], in these groups. Diabetics and epileptics controlled on treatment in hospital may not be well controlled at home and school. Older children can be more closely involved in monitoring their diet and insulin by measuring their blood sugars at home and school using the Ames Eyetone reflectance meter. The school nurse and the paediatric nurse can support and guide these young people in their day to day problems with the help of the paediatrician and the school doctor.

Written instructions should be available in all schools on the management of a seizure or an attack of hypoglycaemia. Understanding of a chronic disorder is needed, not only by the class teacher, but also the child's classmates and other teachers who may come in contact with the child. This need was highlighted by a report from Sweden[37] which showed that many teachers were ignorant of the management and the preceding signs of hypoglycaemia when they had a child with diabetes in their school, and many diabetic children were teased by the other children if they ate a special diet.

obesity

When a child's weight is 20% above the expected weight for his height and age, that child may be said to be obese[38]. The commonest cause of obesity is an excessive intake of food compared with expenditure of energy. A detailed description of the child's eating habits and intake throughout the day as well as the family's pattern of eating needs to be obtained. A simple reduction in calories and if necessary the help of a dietitian in prescribing a suitable diet is the first stage of treatment. Alteration of the family's eating habits may need to be tried. The most difficult cases are those families whose diet consists largely of refined carbohydrate and packaged food, where a major meal of protein would be a pork pie. There are some children who do not eat excessively, although they are obese, and it is extremely difficult for them to lose weight. The handicapped child often has difficulty in maintaining correct weight[39], as after stunted growth and difficulty with feeding in infancy, when appetite is established, even for the wrong food, their grateful parents will encourage overeating. There is a particular problem with Down's syndrome children, who are great lovers of bread and will eat enormous amounts if allowed to do so. Early counselling on diet for parents with a handicapped child is as important as early counselling on discipline. A plump or naughty 3-year-old is tolerable but a rude, badly behaved and obese 14-year-old is very unattractive and will not elicit the help needed by that young man or woman in society.

Although the treatment of obesity can be unrewarding in all age groups[40], regular follow-up and the interest of a sympathetic practitioner, in conjunction with the weight reducing classes run by school nurses and health visitors, can be effective and help to reduce the misery of the fat schoolchild. The longterm ill-effects of obesity are reduced life expectancy and increased life insurance premiums, with an increased risk of hypertension, diabetes mellitus, gall bladder disease, osteoarthritis and complications of surgery[41].

Perthes' disease

During the years in the nursery and the infant school, the school doctor will be asked to see children who limp. Very often this is due to minor injury but in a small proportion of cases the limp is due to the onset of Perthes' disease, which affects 2 children per thousand in the 4 to 7 age group[42]. The child may complain of pain in the knee but careful examination will disclose limitation of movement in the hip, in the early stages limitation of abduction and external rotation of the joint. The disorder is due to a healing infarct of the femoral head epiphysis[43]. The sex ratio is 4 : 1 in favour of boys and one case in ten is bilateral. It is rare in negroes.

Many of the affected children are retarded in skeletal growth and maturation[44], and there appears to be an excess of abnormalities affecting the inguinal region and the genito-urinary tract of patients and their near relatives[45]. Children with Perthes' disease are smaller in every measurement except skull circumference, although a growth spurt occurs later. Children with suspected Perthes' disease should be referred to the orthopaedic clinic. Treatment will depend on the severity of the disease. Most children are rapidly discharged from hospital and returned home in plaster or splints and, with help, many of them will return to their local schools. If the local school find this is difficult, a short period of home teaching may be necessary until the child is more mobile.

dental care

Regular dental inspection of schoolchildren's teeth and the provision of surgical care with an emphasis on conservative management and hygiene are provided by the school dental service. Many children will attend their own dental practitioner for surgical treatment following the dental officer's examination at school. A mobile surgery may be provided for the handicapped children in special schools. Children who are severely mentally handicapped may need hospital dental care if inspection and treatment under a general anaesthetic proves necessary.

learning problems

The child with a sensory handicap needs very close supervision. A review[46] of children with a recognized hearing loss, whether moderate or severe, bilateral or unilateral, showed that visual defects occurred more frequently in this group. The children were often clumsy with speech difficulties, poor expressive language development and low educational attainments not always recognized by their teachers. The children with severe bilateral and unilateral hearing loss showed more disturbed behaviour patterns. It is astounding how well intelligent children with severe speech disorder and/or hearing loss can learn to use another child to interpret and respond for them and so cover up their difficulties in the classroom and at home.

Children who fail appointments, children undergoing treatment or recovering from severe illness and children with a disability will be seen annually at school either by the school doctor or the school nurse. Selective medical examination would be most fruitful in the 7+ age group, before the children move to the junior school. At 7 years of age children who may not be able to learn in the more formal, self-directing atmosphere of the junior school will be more easily recognized. There is a need to counsel the parents of this group of children and to prepare both the children and their parents for a change of school or the need for remedial help at the junior school. Successful counselling of the parents by the health and education staff is the most important factor in the future educational attainment of the child.

Language and thought are said to merge in children between 5 and 8 years of age, and, if this integration does not happen, the child must use a different set of symbols for thinking[47]. Older children and adults use internal speech to memorize verbal material, whether heard or read, but some profoundly deaf children do not do so[48].

Children under 7 years of age perceive whole objects rather than details. They often disregard spatial relationships as they can as easily recognize objects held upside down as upright and fail to distinguish that a shape is inverted. Normal children may continue to have this difficulty in remembering the shapes of letters and distinguishing them from their mirror image, e.g. *b* and *d*, *p* and *q*, *n* and *u*.

How should the doctor assess the child with a learning problem? Having attempted to elucidate the part played by other factors such as family history, sibling rivalry, and the presence or absence of a sensory handicap in the examination of the child, one should look at the child's school work, namely their reading and writing book. Little children will often come to the school doctor with their work books: if not, the doctor should arrange to see them. Some parents will firmly believe that their child can read when he can't, or will say that they have been worried for some time about their child's failure to learn and that the child's teacher has failed to teach the child properly. These parental reactions are to be treated sympathetically while not undermining the work of the child's teacher.

One can demonstrate that the child can 'read' his reading book but not the same words in other books. School doctors will use their favourite children's book as a test of reading ability or an accepted reading scale, such as the Holborn reading scale[49] which tests reading ages from 5 years 9 months to 13 years 9 months, using sentences rather than individual words. With the reading difficulties of the 7+ age group, the first sentence is all one needs. The sentence reads 'The dog got wet and Tom had to rub him dry'. The child may only recognize one or two simple words such as 'the', 'and', 'to'. The doctor is not testing the child's intelligence and must not commit the child to failure in order to demonstrate to the parents the child's problem. This is the first step in counselling and is a prelude to the more expert help and guidance that will be made available by the psychologist. The child is helped as much as is necessary to read the sentence and the help given is utilized by the doctor to obtain an estimate of the child's innate ability. Proceed through the sentence until the last phrase when the difficult word 'rub' occurs. Ask the child 'how would Tom dry his dog?', or, if that is outside the child's experience, 'how does mummy dry your hair?' The average child will give the correct answer.

If an assessment of numeracy is needed, the child may be asked to count to five using bricks or the earpieces of the auriscope. When the child has counted the five pieces, ask him to place in your hand two or three of them. Don't stop the child if he returns all five. If the correct number is returned this will demonstrate not only an ability to count but that the child understands number to two or three. More complicated testing should be done under proper test conditions by a psychologist.

Education in British schools depends on a child learning to be literate and numerate. The four main psychological processes involved in learning to read are – intelligence, motivation, visual perception and audio-linguistic perception[50].

A study of 1900 children undertaken between 1966 and 1969 showed that 6% of children after 3 years at school needed help with basic reading skills[51]. Reading difficulties found in children in the 7+ age group should be reviewed and referred to the school psychological service, who will provide either a formal assessment of the problem and/or the support of the specialist teaching service.

A typical example is the case of Guy who was referred to the Child Guidance Clinic at the age of 7 years with reading difficulty. He had normal vision, hearing, physical and neurological development. His teacher thought he had normal potential, although he had not made a start in reading, had become very frustrated and was developing behaviour problems. When seen by the psychologist, Guy was found to be of normal intelligence with an oral vocabulary above average. His grasp of instructions was above average and he was quite articulate. He had had considerable individual help with reading at school but despite this his reading age on the Neale test[52] was nil. There were two older boys in the family who had had similar problems and had improved. The parents were most helpful and co-operative. It was decided to give Guy a period of intensive help at the Child Guidance Clinic to supplement that already being given at school. Three years later Guy is in the remedial group at his junior school. He has progressed and has a mechanical reading age of 7.11 on the Neale test. He has great difficulty in differentiating the similarities and differences within and between spoken words, illustrated by his spelling problems, e.g. 'god' for 'guard'. His copy writing has greatly improved. Although Guy is well supported at home and school, he is still tense and anxious when asked to read and write.

The two categories of reading difficulty, as defined by Rutter and Yule[53], are:

(1) *Reading backwardness.* These children have a low attainment on reading accuracy or comprehension on the Neale Test of Reading Ability. All these children have an IQ below average.

(2) *Specific reading retardation.* These children have a low attainment on reading accuracy or comprehension on the Neale Test although the children have an

average intelligence quotient.

Investigation of these two groups of children in the Isle of Wight study[30] showed that the children with reading backwardness have an even sex distribution and a high incidence of overt neurological disorder such as cerebral palsy. The children show delay in neurological development with poor motor co-ordination. Motor impersistence, that is an inability to sustain a voluntary motor act initiated by a verbal command, poor right–left differentiation, difficulty in making or drawing shapes (a triangle, mental age 6 years; or a diamond, mental age 7 years), speech delay and language impairment were also more common in this group. The children were from large families and their fathers were employed in unskilled work.

Specific reading retardation on the other hand is more common in boys, the sex ratio being 3 : 1 boys to girls. Overt neurological disorder is uncommon but there is frequently a delay in speech and language development. The disorder is commoner in children of large families but there is no social class differentiation. In both groups, there is a positive family history of speech delay or reading difficulty in the siblings or the parents, the incidence being three times higher than in the general population.

The groups were reassessed after 4–5 years[54]. The reading retarded children had made significantly less progress than the children with reading backwardness both in reading accuracy and spelling, whereas the reading retarded group had made more progress in the arithmetic–mathematics tests than the reading backward.

dyslexia

Dyslexia means word blindness. The term 'specific developmental dyslexia' is defined as a disorder manifested by difficulty in learning to read despite conventional instruction, adequate intelligence and socio-cultural opportunity. It is dependent upon fundamental cognitive disabilities which are frequently of constitutional origin[55]. This definition has been criticized as lacking in clarity[53]. The characteristics of dyslexia described in the literature as significant of cognitive disability are also features of specific reading retardation especially the speech and language problems. Mixed handedness which is described as a feature has been shown by epidemiological studies[30,56] not to be so. It would seem sensible to define reading difficulties in children as either reading backwardness or specific reading retardation and not to use the term dyslexia.

gifted children

Children with exceptional ability and talent may show evidence of this at an early age – by needing less sleep in infancy, early language development and early reading ability. The children may be regarded by their parents and siblings as a nuisance, or as overactive, but not uselessly so, and excessively questioning. Further evidence will become apparent to the skilled teacher. The gifted child's need for educational advantage should be assisted and encouraged by all professionals working with children with understanding of the family's problems. Gifted children are those who show consistently remarkable performance in any worthwhile endeavour[57]. These children usually have outstanding personality characteristics, such as commonsense, a sense of humour, conscientiousness, self-confidence and truthfulness[58]. As well as an extensive vocabulary, they have good powers of comprehension, observation, reasoning, memory and relational thinking.

In education, one must distinguish between the child with unusual or specific abilities such as in music, mathematics or the arts and the child with high general intellectual ability. Special schools are available in these fields. The management of the child with high general ability is not so easy. There is considerable controversy over whether there should be special schools for this group of children, the children given more skilled teaching in the local school, or placed in a higher class in keeping with their intellectual ability rather than their chronological age. The children may suffer emotionally if they are not recognized and stimulated as they have the same emotional needs as other children but may not be acceptable to older, larger children as friends. Neglect or ridicule at home or school with lack of friends will cause such a child considerable distress and cause him to repress his gifts so as to be acceptable to his elders and his peers. Further advice and counselling can be obtained by parents and teachers and other interested professionals from the National Association for Gifted Children.

references

1. Education Act, 1944. (London: HMSO)
2. Kellmer Pringle, M. L., Butler, N. R. and Davie, R. (1969). *11000 Seven-year-olds – The National Child Development Study.* (London: Longman)
3. Wood, M. E. (1973). *Children: The Development of Personality and Behaviour.* (London: Harrap)
4. Moore, T. (1966). Difficulties of the ordinary child in adjusting to primary school. *J. Child Psychol. Psychiatry*, **7**, 17
5. Piaget, J. (1932). *The Moral Judgement of the Child.* (London: Routledge and Kegan Paul)
6. Special Educational Needs: Report of the Committee of Enquiry into the Education of Handicapped Children and Young People. (1978). (London: HMSO)
7. Bamford, F. N. (1977). The school health service: methods. In Mitchell, R. G. *Child Health in the Community.* (Edinburgh: Churchill Livingstone)
8. Webb, L. (1967). *Children with Special Needs in Infants' Schools.* (London: Smythe)
9. Bailey, V., Graham, P. and Boniface, D. (1978). How much child psychiatry does a general practitioner do? *J. R. Coll. Gen. Practit.*, **28**, 621
10. Editorial (1977). On Pissing in the Bedde – and elsewhere. *Lancet*, **2**, 1214
11. Rolleston, G. L., Maling, T. M. H. and Hodson, C. J. (1974). Intrarenal reflux and the scarred kidney. *Arch. Dis. Child.*, **49**, 531
12. Smellis, J. M. *et al.* (1976). Long term low dose co-trimoxazole in prophylaxis of childhood urinary tract infection: clinical aspects. *Br. Med. J.*, **2**, 203
13. Cardiff–Oxford Bacteriuria Study Group (1978). Sequelae of covert bacteriuria in schoolgirls. *Lancet*, **1**, 889
14. Lindberg, U. (1978). Asymptomatic bacteriuria in schoolgirls. VIII. Clinical course during a 3-year follow-up. *J. Paediatr.*, **92,** 194

15. Smellie, J. M. and Normand, I. C. S. (1975). Bacteriuria, reflux and renal scarring. *Arch. Dis. Child.*, **50**, 581
16. Berg, I., Fielding, D. and Meadow, S. R. (1977). Psychiatric disturbance, urgency and bacteriuria in children with day and night wetting. *Arch. Dis. Child.*, **52**, 651
17. Turner, K. R. (1973). Conditioning treatment of nocturnal enuresis: present status. In Kolvin, I., MacKeith, R. C. and Meadow, S. R. (eds.) *Bladder Control and Enuresis.* (London & Philadelphia: Heinemann)
18. Dische, S. (1973). Treatment of enuresis with an enuresis alarm. In Kolvin, I., MacKeith, R. C., and Meadow, S. R. (eds.) *Bladder Control and Enuresis.* (London & Philadelphia: Heinemann)
19. Meadow, S. R. (1977). How to use buzzer alarms to cure bed wetting. *Br. Med. J.*, **2**, 1073
20. *From Birth to Seven*: the second report of the National Child Development Study (1958 cohort) (1972). (London: Longman)
21. Clayden, G. S. (1976). Constipation and soiling in childhood. *Br. Med. J.* **1**, 515
22. Berg, I. and Jones, K. V. (1964). Functional faecal incontinence in children. *Arch. Dis. Child.*, **39**, 465
23. Clayden, G. S. and Lawson, J. O. N. (1976). Investigation and management of long-standing chronic constipation in childhood. *Arch. Dis. Child.*, **51**, 918
24. Lawson, J. O. N. and Nixon, H. H. J. (1967). Anal canal pressures in the diagnosis of Hirschsprung's disease. *J. Paediatr. Surg.*, **2**, 544
25. Kornfalt, R. and Kohler, L. (1978). Physical health of ten-year-old children. *Acta Paediatr. Scand.*, **67**, 481
26. Jacoby, N. M. (1966). Steroid treatment of asthmatic children. *Lancet*, **2**, 1354
27. Blair, H. (1977). Natural history of childhood asthma: 20-year follow-up. *Arch. Dis. Child.*, **52**, 613
28. Sims, D. G. *et al.* (1976). Respiratory syncytial virus infection in north-east England. *Br. Med. J.*, **2**, 1095
29. Gulliford, R. (1971). *Special Educational Needs.* (London: Routledge and Kegan Paul)
30. Rutter, M., Tizard, J. and Whitmore, K. (1970). *Education, Health and Behaviour.* (London: Longman)
31. Stores, G., Hart, J. and Piran, N. (1978). Inattentiveness in schoolchildren with epilepsy. *Epilepsia*, **19**, 169
32. Pond, D. A. and Espir, M. (1978). Epilepsy. In Raffle, A. (ed.) *Medical Aspects of Fitness to Drive.* (London: Dorriston)
33. White, F. A. (1976). *Widening Horizons of Child Health.* (Lancaster: MTP Press)
34. DHSS. (1971). *Hospital Facilities for Children* HM(71)22. (London: HMSO)
35. Sorsby, A. (1966). *Incidence and Causes of Blindness in England and*

Wales. (London: HMSO)

36. MacGregor, M. (1977). Juvenile diabetics growing up. *Lancet*, **1**, 943
37. Ludwigsson, J. (1977). Diabetics in school: knowledge and attitudes of school staff in relation to juvenile diabetics. *Scand. J. Med.*, **5**, 21
38. Lloyd, J. K., Wolff, O. H. and Whelan, N. S. (1961). Childhood obesity. *Br. Med. J.*, **2**, 146
39. Guy, R. (1978). The growth of physically handicapped children with emphasis on appetite and activity. *Public Health*, **92**, 145
40. Bruch, H. (1971). Modern Perspectives. In Howels, J. G. (ed.) *Adolescent Psychiatry*. (Edinburgh: Oliver and Boyd)
41. Kannel, W. B. *et al.* (1967). Relation of body weight to development of coronary heart disease. *Circulation*, **35**, 734
42. Editorial (1978). Clues in Perthes's disease. *Br. Med. J.*, **2**, 231
43. Jensen, O. M. and Lauritzen, J. (1976). Legg–Calve–Perthes disease. Morphological studies in two cases examined at necropsy. *J. Bone Jt. Surg.*, **58B**, 332
44. Harrison, M. H. M., Turner, M. H. and Jacobs, P. (1976). Skeletal immaturity in Perthes disease. *J. Bone Jt. Surg.*, **58B**, 37
45. Catterall, A., Lloyd-Roberts, G. C. and Wynn-Davies, R. (1971). Association of Perthes' disease with congenital anomalies of the genito-urinary tract and inguinal region. *Lancet*, **1**, 996
46. Peckham, C. S., Sheridan, M. and Butler, N. R. (1972). School attainment of seven-year-old children with hearing difficulties. *Devel. Med. Child Neurol.*, **14**, 592
47. Vygotsky, L. S. (1962). *Thought and Language*. (New York and London: John Wiley and Sons)
48. Medical Research Council Annual Report (1973). *Cognitive Deficits in Children*. (London: HMSO)
49. Watts, A. F. (1944). *The Holborn Reading Scale*. (London: Harrap)
50. Vernon, M. D. (1971). *Reading and Its Difficulties: a Psychological Study*. (Cambridge: Cambridge University Press)
51. Clark, M. M. (1970). *Reading Difficulties in Schools*. (Harmondsworth: Penguin Books)
52. Neale, M. D. (1958). *Neale Analysis of Reading Ability Manual*. (London: Macmillan)
53. Rutter, M. and Yule, W. (1975). The concept of specific reading retardation. *J. Child Psychol. Psychiatry*, **16**, 181
54. Yule, W. (1973). Differential prognosis of reading backwardness and specific reading retardation. *Br. J. Educ. Psychol.*, **43**, 244
55. Critchley, M. (1970). *The Dyslexic Child*. (Springfield, Illinois: Thomas)
56. Malmquist, E. (1958). *Factors related to Reading Disabilities in the First Grade of Elementary School*. (Stockholm: Almquist and Witskell)
57. Terman, L. M. (1926). *Mental and Physical Traits of a Thousand*

Gifted Children in Genetic Studies of Genius. (Stanford: Stanford University Press)

58. Parkyn, G. W. (1949). *Children with High Intelligence*. (London: Oxford University Press)

chapter six

the years from 7 to 12

8 to 12 years

This period of a child's life is aptly described as the period of latency with a change from the egocentricity of childhood to an awareness and an understanding of the feelings of others[1]. It is a period of calm and concentration on work and play. There is less illness and fewer accidents. Between 8 and 11 years of age, children develop permanent attitudes to work, make friends and discover how popular they are and whether they are as clever as their peers[2].

By 9 years of age, children will understand mood and will note personal physical characteristics[3]. With increasing cognitive ability children will use deduction to explain behaviour and will use language to express ideas but not feelings. By 10 years of age, children will consider a person's attitude to others as well as themselves when making judgements. Play now becomes more complex with co-operation in playing games and a willingness to alter the rules if other players are agreed. Thus children develop mutual respect and consideration for the rights of others[4].

Regardless of sex, most children have a preference for their mother but wish to resemble the parent of the same sex[5]. At 7 to 9 years of age, children enjoy joint activities with their parents. By 10 to 12 years, children are more aware of the presence or absence of discipline by their parents and their teachers and show less need for joint activities. The 8- to 11-year-olds note bad temper, unfairness and excessive strictness in their parents and, like the younger children, are distressed by shouting. They will judge what they regard to be unfair behaviour on the part of other adults, which may be illustrated by the story of a delightful, clever lad. His father was unemployed and involved in minor crime, as were his older brothers. Two of his brothers in the senior school took their younger brother with them when breaking into a factory. The younger boy, unable to reach the escape window, was caught by the police and remanded by the magistrates for three weeks. A remand, in his experience, had never happened to his older brothers, and from being a delightful person, the boy returned to school sullen and resentful, full of anger and misery. With such an unsupportive family, the chances of helping this boy to recover and to achieve his high educational potential are doubtful.

The child from a linguistically deprived background will become more severely handicapped as the teaching of subjects requires more complex expressive speech. Language is necessary for clear and logical thought and the linguistically deprived child will find increasing difficulty in understanding fully the range of lessons offered and will show an inability to express himself with clarity[6]. These problems are compounded when there are changes of home and school.

Thoughtful parents consider their children's educational advantage as far as possible when changes have to be made for work and/or a new home. Deprived children will frequently come from homes where, to avoid debt or due to the instability of the marriage, the children are subject to changes of housing and school. These changes may be associated with a general inability on the part of the parents to understand or their lack of concern for their own future and that of their children, increasing their children's disadvantage. Social workers, before recommending changes of home for problem families, should consult medical and education staff who may know and have had longer contact with the family concerned. Neighbours are also an important part of the family's environment. Where the neighbours have learned to tolerate the difficult and feckless family, the children of that family are relieved of a burden and may grow and develop with less shame and misery. The latter symptoms become more noticeable in junior age children, as they become aware of the differences in the care they receive from their parents compared with their peers.

Children who transfer from special schools or other establishments to ordinary schools may present particular problems or learning difficulties. Three children here illustrated show the importance of an attractive personality with their classmates and their teachers plus drive, intelligence and/or special gifts in succeeding against the odds. These children all have serious handicaps, physical and social.

The first child, Karen, prior to adoption, had been in a children's home and attended a school for physically handicapped children. She was known to have above average intelligence and marked behaviour difficulties. Her adoptive parents had known her for some time and were convinced that she could respond to a normal home and an ordinary school. The child had abnormal upper limbs in the shape of two flippers, which she was able to use for writing and painting, and she could manage toileting, feeding and dressing but not difficult fastenings. The local primary school, which her adopted brother and sister attended, agreed to admit Karen. The school doctor and the psychologist had visited the school, and would continue to do so intermittently, to ensure that there were no serious problems of adaptation and behaviour. Initially, there were minor behaviour problems and some reading difficulties which needed specialist help, but the settling in process went surprisingly smoothly. There may be more difficult problems when this girl reaches adolescence so continuous follow-up will be needed.

The second child, David, had a history of deprivation since infancy. As a small boy of 4 years, he was referred to the child guidance clinic with a behaviour problem. The family were rehoused and David attended the local infant school who reported no serious difficulties. At 10 years of age, he was referred to the child psychiatrist and the paediatrician with impulsive behaviour, inattention, lack of concentration and retarded social development with evident clumsiness. His hearing and vision were normal. His school report described him as a chatterbox with little concentration. His handwriting and mathematics were poor and he appeared to have difficulty with spatial relationships. He is merry, sensitive, very kind and in composition he showed considerable imagination. The paediatrician could find no evidence of epilepsy. David showed poor co-ordination in fine motor movement but no abnormal neurological signs. Physiotherapy would be helpful in teaching him how to co-ordinate his body and limb movements. Careful consideration will be needed in the choice of senior school for David. A small unit would appear to be the most suitable choice. Teaching him to use an electric typewriter might usefully improve David's handwriting. This may alleviate much of his clumsiness in handling a pen and pencil and may also be a means of harnessing his gift for imaginative storywriting.

The third child, Betty, was the illegitimate daughter of a young, immature woman who deserted her baby within a few weeks of birth. Betty had multiple congenital abnormalities and feeding difficulties. An attempt to give the child a longterm foster home failed, probably for the same reason that the mother deserted. At the age of 2 years, she was admitted to a hospital for the mentally subnormal for care and treatment. Here first-stage plastic surgery was started and it became apparent that the child was not as retarded as first thought. From the hospital, Betty was transferred to a combined home and school. By the age of 7 years, the head of the home was confident that this little girl had quite considerable ability and arranged for a senior educational psychologist to see her, who, on testing, found Betty to have normal potential. She was seen by the senior school doctor and arrangements made to complete the plastic surgery. The doctor and the psychologist agreed to try to arrange through the authorities concerned, i.e. the Local Social Services and the Local Education Authority, for Betty to be fostered (Social Services) and to be admitted to an ordinary school (Education).

There was some delay in these arrangements and it was reported that Betty was regressing socially and educationally at her children's home. A foster home was not possible so she was admitted to an ordinary children's home and the local primary school. Betty was delighted with both her children's home and her new school. She took part in all activities, made friends and showed considerable social confidence, although there were minor episodes of aggressive behaviour. Her school report shows that her written work is better than her oral work and she shows talent in both design and colour. Her drawings always include a house. Plastic surgery is not yet complete. When it is, further attempts will be made to find this delightful child a permanent home and family.

chronic disabilities

In all cases of chronic disability, whether the children are being educated in ordinary or special schools, the child and the parents need to understand the implications of the disability, what aids or medicines are needed to control the effects of the disorder and the changes that may occur with growth. Clear instructions need to be given to the child, the parents and the teaching staff regarding any precautions that may be necessary in physical education and sport.

dental health

Continuing attention to dental hygiene by attention to diet and gum massage with tooth brushing should be stressed. Orthodontic treatment for malocclusion usually starts between 11 and 12 years of age[7], as earlier treatment is not beneficial due to variations in growth and eruption of teeth and may actually prolong the need for treatment[8].

Referral for orthodontic treatment is made by the child's dental practitioner and regular dental treatment is necessary. Both School Health Dental Services and Hospital Dental Services run orthodontic clinics.

health education

Most area health authorities have specialist departments of health education which provide pamphlets, films and other material and also run courses on good health practice and the prevention of illness for any service involved in education in the broadest sense.

Between 8 and 11 years of age, when children are ready for work and learning, the school nurse has an invaluable role to play in reinforcing good health practice as well as the prevention of bad habits, such as smoking and alcohol abuse. The teaching staff can incorporate the nurse's advice into various lessons; the parents can use the advice in the general health and care of themselves and their children, not forgetting advice on the buying and preparation of food especially for immigrant mothers and for those who are not capable at managing a budget; and by her regular observation and contact with the children themselves, there is an opportunity for the nurse to talk to individual children or small groups of children about eating habits, cleanliness and regular dental care, to an audience who admire and respect her and who are receptive to teaching.

Dental hygienists also give regular talks and displays at schools on teeth cleaning and good eating habits. Learning about health, behaviour, family and social relationships is an integral part of the daily life both at home and at school and is best introduced to children at school as part of the general curriculum, not as a specialist subject[9]. Both the school doctor and the school nurse by their contact with teachers, parents and children have an important role to play in improving the general health of the community.

references

1. Winnicott, D. W. (1965). *The Maturational Processes and the Facilitating Environment.* (London: Hogarth Press)
2. Erikson, E. H. (1965). *Childhood and Society.* (Harmondsworth: Penguin Books)
3. Wood, M. (1973). *Children: the Development of Personality and Behaviour.* (London: Harrap)
4. Piaget, J. (1951). *Play, Dreams and Imitation in Childhood.* (New York: Norton)
5. Kagan, J. (1956). The child's perception of the parent. *J. Abnorm. Soc. Psychol.*, **53**, 257
6. Hawkes, G. R. and Pease, D. (1962). *Behaviour and Development from Five to Twelve.* (New York: Harper and Row)
7. Todd, J. E. (1975). *Children's Dental Health in England and Wales.* (London: HMSO)
8. Lieberman, M. A. and Gazit, E. J. (1974). Guides to orthodontic treatment timing. *J. Am. Dent. Assoc.*, **88**, 555
9. Winnicott, D. W. (1957). *The Child and the Outside World.* (London: Tavistock Publications)

chapter seven

adolescence

normal development

Adolescence is generally understood to be that period of life between puberty and adulthood. Puberty is characterized by a growth spurt in height and muscular development, with an alteration in the shape of the sexes, rapid development of the gonads and the genitalia and the appearance of secondary sexual characteristics. As well as an increase in musculature, there is an increase in the size and the weight of the heart and rapid growth of the lungs with a decline in basal metabolism[1].

The range of development of children of the same age shows wide variation, the growth spurt of girls beginning two years in advance of boys. For girls, the average age for the growth spurt is 11 to 12 years and for boys 13 to 14 years, with a wide variability of development in girls of 11, 12 and 13 years and boys of 13, 14 and 15 years.

The age of appearance of the secondary sexual characteristics also varies. In girls, the appearance of breast buds usually precedes the growth of pubic hair, growth of the vagina and the uterus occurring *pari passu* with the development of the breasts. The menarche occurs late after the peak in growth rate has passed although further growth may occur. In boys, the earliest changes are in the growth of the testes and the scrotum followed by the growth of pubic hair. Growth of the penis accompanies the spurt in height, followed about two years later by the development of axillary and facial hair, breaking of the voice and the first seminal discharge.

In girls one breast bud may appear earlier or be more prominent than the other and boys may develop gynaecomastia which lasts about a year. Both these signs are normal. If a pupil, found with these at a routine medical inspection, does not mention them, the doctor should do so with reassurance. Details of the limits of adolescent pubertal development are obtainable[2,3]. Girls worry most about the delay in the appearance of the menarche and the irregularity of their menstrual periods after the menarche. In the older adolescent the most common problem is heavy or painful periods, most handicapping at the time of examinations. Undoubtedly stress plays a part but a small proportion of girls are seriously disabled by painful and/or heavy periods and need expert management. Boys mostly worry about their height and growth. Knowledge of the relationship of the peak in growth rate to pubertal development is essential. Care in excluding pathology in both these groups is needed, e.g. the amenorrhoea of anorexia nervosa needs to be differentiated from the temporary cessation of periods after the menarche. The majority of adolescents are well able to cope with their growing sexuality[4].

school medical problems

One of the commonest problems in the adolescent is acne. Whilst this is troublesome and requires scrupulous and regular attention to cleanliness, exercise and diet, the response of the more disfiguring form of acne in both boys and girls to longterm tetracycline therapy is excellent. Tetracycline used in this way has been a powerful agent of good mental health.

Of the orthopaedic anomalies, scoliosis is the most common and most important. Many diseases can cause spinal curvature, congenital abnormalities of the vertebrae, myopathy and neuropathy but the most common form of scoliosis is the idiopathic variety occurring mainly in adolescent girls. The incidence is not certain, although a survey in Edinburgh[5] found an occurrence rate of 4 : 1000 girls, nor is it known if there is any difference in incidence between ethnic groups. When examining for scoliosis, the whole spine should be visible and palpated, both in the upright position and in forward flexion. Referral to the paediatric orthopaedic clinic with early treatment, physiotherapy and splintage may prevent surgery. There is a familial basis to idiopathic scoliosis, with thirty times the expected frequency of incidence occurring in first degree relatives[5]. The untreated or ineffectively treated outcome is grave physical handicap and early death[6,7].

Slipped femoral epiphysis, although uncommon, occurs more commonly in boys and needs urgent referral to the orthopaedic clinic. The patient presents with similar symptoms and signs to Perthes' disease, i.e. pain often referred to the knee with limitation of abduction and external rotation of the hip joint. Osteochondritis of the tibial tubercle, the calcaneum or the vertebral epiphysis is also uncommon but occur in adolescents, giving rise to pain and disability, and should be referred to the orthopaedic clinic. Chondromalacia patellae is somewhat more common and gives rise to local pain which is reproduced by manipulation of the patella. The pain and disability may last for a year. The only treatment necessary is to limit activities such as sport and cycling, and prolonged kneeling for those pupils whose religious observance demands such activity.

Accidents become more common as a cause of death and morbidity in the adolescent with a sharp rise in road traffic accidents in the 14+ age group. Head injuries are not uncommon and may cause considerable individual disturbance on return to school where recovery is incomplete or where sequelae have altered the pupil's concentration, learning ability or behaviour.

Head injuries are divided into minor and severe[8]. Minor head injury is an injury causing post-traumatic amnesia of less than 24 hours or requiring less than seven days admission to hospital. Severe head injury is one where the duration of amnesia was longer, the length of stay in hospital was longer or where the skull was fractured. If the injured person cannot remember the blow to the head, then he is considered to have been concussed – there has been loss of consciousness however brief[9]. All pupils with head injury should be followed up at school to alleviate excessive tiredness which may result in irritability, although this is more likely following concussion and/or severe head injury. Students of 15 to 20 years return to school or further education earlier than the same age group return to work, 5.6 days compared with 7.6 days. If pupils have had a head injury, physical education teachers should be advised that precautions must be taken not to allow these pupils to take undue risks as the effects of concussion are cumulative and have permanent sequelae consequent upon neuronal loss[10].

A final medical examination will be carried out on selected pupils at 14 years of age. For the assistance of the Careers Advisory Officer, a medical certificate will be completed on all pupils on the basis of previous medical examinations and routine screening procedures. A more detailed certificate, countersigned by the parent, is completed on handicapped pupils for the Careers Advisory Service and the Employment Medical Advisory Service (EMAS).

psychological development and emotional changes

As part of the physical and sexual changes in adolescence there comes a complex psychological reorientation – the adolescent search for independence, with separation from childhood and a loosening of the ties with their parents, as well as the development of control over their emerging sexuality and assertiveness – culminating in the achievement of an adult identity[11].

Most adolescents and their parents cope with these moves to independence. In a survey of 14-year-olds[12], apart from minor disagreements with their parents over clothes, appearance and social outings, alienation from parents was not common in this age group, but is probably more common in late teens. Young people tend to share their parents' values and respect the need for control.

Social pressures from other adults and the peer group also play a substantial role in the behaviour of the adolescent. Teachers and other adults may expect change before the adolescent is ready. This altered expectation produces stress and would appear to be related to our social values. This type of stress on the adolescent is less apparent in other cultures[13]. The need to conform to the standards of behaviour of the peer group is often a cause of disagreements with the parents[14].

Changes in the schoolroom, with the aim of encouraging 'initiative, independence and creativity', have wrought changes in the pupils, and, whereas adults tend to approve of the questioning, discursive child in the junior school, they are less happy dealing with the more verbal and critical adolescent[15].

From 12 years of age, children are able to think in terms of the possible and not only the actual. By 13 years of age, they are able to use inference, conjecture and speculation to understand behaviour with further development of logical reasoning[4]. There is no increase in IQ but cognitive abilities such as reasoning, creativity and mathematical skills improve.

Psychiatric disturbance is slightly more common in adolescence and may be divided into two groups – that due to transient symptoms and that due to persistent symptoms[16]. In the Isle of Wight study, about 25% of the parents reported communication difficulties with their sons although this problem was not new. Communication difficulties were less frequent with girls[17].

Feelings of misery and depression were reported by 20% of the boys and girls, with difficulty in sleeping and early waking, and were accompanied by feelings of self-depreciation. Although a cause of pain to the adolescent these feelings frequently went unrecognized by the adults around them[12].

Persistent symptoms causing frank psychiatric disorder occurred in 7.5% of the 14-year-olds[12], and would probably be much higher in an urban population as was found in a comparative study of 10-year-olds[17]. The types of disorder found are the same as those which occur in childhood, neurotic and conduct disorders, which may be mixed, and psychotic illness, which is rare in early adolescence[2]. Depression and school refusal are more common than in childhood, the presence of depression showing a shift towards the adult type of disorder, but there is not the marked adult preponderance of females to males as conduct disorders are more common in boys.

Many adolescent psychiatric conditions are a continuation of childhood disorders. They are more common in boys and associated with disturbed family backgrounds, alienation from parents and educational difficulties – whether due to mental handicap or lack of opportunity to learn from truancy[12]. Psychiatric disorder arising *de novo* in adolescence has an equal sex incidence, affecting young people from stable homes without educational difficulties, but associated with parental alienation which began in childhood.

Sexual problems concerning masturbation and heterosexual and homosexual relationships are more common in these groups. The increased incidence of depression leads to a rise in the suicide rate and suicide may be a consequence of parental death[18]. These young people will sometimes exhibit their unhappiness by attending the school clinic with innumerable minor ailments or with a neighbour's younger children and it may be two or three weeks before they can express their underlying fears and anxiety.

The prognosis in all disorders depends on the diagnosis rather than the age of onset[12].

Anorexia nervosa is symptomatic of severe psychiatric illness and requires urgent admission to hospital.

Drug addiction tends to vary widely from hard drugs to glue sniffing, the current adult concern being the rising consumption of alcohol and smoking. Two studies in France[19,20] showed that a campaign against smoking was well received, largely because of appreciation of the effect on others as pollution and on pregnancy, but most young people do not feel concerned about alcoholism[20], although alcoholism is a serious cause of chronic illhealth in adults. Children are more likely to smoke if their parents smoke[21]. Where there is evidence of illegal drugs being used, the police drug squad should be informed and are extremely helpful.

psychiatric clinics

Difficulties may arise for the school doctor with a rising school leaving age and the treatment of older adolescents in adult psychiatric clinics. There is less co-operation by adult psychiatrists with the school medical service than exists with child psychiatrists. This lack of communication may cause problems where school attendance is a major factor and the school doctor is responsible for advising the parents and teaching staff about the educational needs, and the local education authority about its statutory obligations concerning the patient.

contraception, abortion and pregnancy

Contraceptive advice and treatment is available from family doctors, the Family Planning Association (FPA) and other non-health-service agencies such as the Brook Clinics. The alteration in moral values, enabling young men and women to cohabit freely and to marry at 16 years without their parents consent, has increased the need for these services. Girls from disturbed family backgrounds have a high rate of extramarital pregnancy[22] and not uncommonly use their pregnancy and the possibility of abortion as a bargaining counter with the adults with whom they come into contact. Abortion is regarded by many people and particularly by this group of girls as a form of contraception – 7 pregnancies in every 10 in girls under 15 years of age are terminated, usually in the National Health Service hospitals. The pregnancy rate and hence the abortion rate in this group has risen[23] from approximately 3000 in 1970 to 5000 in 1975. Girls from disturbed homes are more likely to truant, and not receive the education necessary to prevent pregnancy, and are often badly cared for, on a poor diet and sleeping rough. 'God help all children as they move into a time of life they do not understand and must struggle through with precepts they have picked from the garbage cans of older people, clinging with the passion of the lost to the odds and ends that will mess them up for all time, or hating the trash so much they will waste their future on the hatred.'[24]

Counselling should be made available before a decision to have an abortion is taken and also following the outcome[25]. The longterm psychological effects on schoolgirls of having a baby or a termination are not known. If a schoolgirl goes on with her pregnancy, either education continues at the girl's school or she has home teaching. The latter may take the form of special classes for small groups of pregnant girls in clinics or other available premises, or the girl may have teaching in her own home or her teacher's home. Teaching the girl in her own home is the least suitable as it is lonely for the girl and divorces her from her friends and company when she is most in need of friendship. After delivery, the girls should be encouraged to return to school. The baby will often be cared for by the maternal grandmother but, if this is not possible, arrangements can be made for the baby to be admitted to a day nursery while the mother is at school. Some education authorities give more extensive teaching in child care, budgeting and general housecraft for these young mothers when they return to school.

counselling

Before leaving school, pupils with congenital and hereditary handicaps need advice on understanding the cause of their handicap, the likely outcome for themselves of the life expectancy of their handicap and the effect of their handicap on their spouses and children if they decide to marry and wish to have children. Handicapped young men and women continue to mix socially after leaving school in clubs and associations and are likely to marry each other. Handicapped pupils with central nervous system disorder need guidance on sexual problems from a doctor who knows about the sexual problems in these disorders and who knows how to advise these pupils.

How far investigation and information on genetic disorders should be undertaken as a routine for all pupils must await society's acknowledgement and understanding of the issues involved but doctors should take the lead in promoting the discussion. It has been suggested that there is a substantial and selective advantage in being a heterozygote and parents should be advised of this advantage[26]. The number of abortions carried out[27] annually on eugenic grounds is 3000. These abortions are legal where, in the opinion of two doctors in good faith, there would be a substantial risk that 'if the child were born it would suffer from such physical or mental abnormalities as to be seriously handicapped'[30]. The Abortion Act protects doctors from the criminal law but does not develop the necessary policy for the nation in view of the public and private interests at stake when selective abortion is used as a means of genetic control[27].

preventive medicine

accidents

The prevention of mortality and morbidity from accidents should take high priority in the education of the adolescent as the incidence of such disasters rises both from motor vehicles and from outdoor sports. Powered motor vehicles, especially motor cycles, are most potent causes of death and serious injury to the brain and spinal cord in adolescents[28]. The wearing of protective helmets is compulsory in the United Kingdom[29]. Care is needed in choosing and replacing the plastic face shields attached to the helmets as some of these shields shatter in accidents, thus causing severe facial and eye injuries, while other shields when scratched make visibility almost nil in oncoming headlight glare and rain. Protective helmets are also needed in other activities such as horse riding and rock climbing.

Classes in road safety are given in all schools and in addition some senior schools give instruction in driving and the maintenance of motor vehicles to boys and to girls. Many senior pupils, with their parents' permission, are encouraged by their schools and education authorities to take part in schemes involving danger and heavy expenditure of energy. It is necessary for the school doctor to ensure that each pupil taking part in these pursuits is fit to do so. The most careful consideration should be given to the precautions necessary for those pupils with epilepsy and diabetes, both to ensure that they are allowed to take part and that the staff involved and the young people themselves are fully informed of these precautions so as not to behave in a foolhardy manner and endanger themselves and the rest of the party.

immunization

Since 1953, vaccination against tuberculosis has been offered to all pupils in the United Kingdom found to have a negative or grade I reaction to tuberculin. Good protection does not always occur with BCG as strains differ in potency[30], although in the British trials the Glaxo strain derived from the Copenhagen strain showed high protective efficacy and is now used routinely in the UK[31]. About 80% protection of the population vaccinated is said to occur with BCG and this level of protection continued throughout the national trials. In India, BCG is given without prior testing with tuberculin to ensure administration and protection of the population against tuberculosis. BCG also produces some protection against leprosy[32].

The incidence of tubercle in adolescents and adults has declined in the United Kingdom, most European countries and the United States of America[33]. The need to continue population vaccination on a large scale is under consideration and the cost effectiveness has been investigated[34]. If routine vaccination were to cease, it would be necessary to continue the vaccination of the population 'at risk' as well as the tracing, investigation and follow-up of contacts.

Since 1968 in the UK immunization against rubella with a live rubella vaccine has been offered to all girls below the age of 14 years. In the USA rubella immunization is offered to all children early in childhood with the hope of eliminating the virus reservoir. The European policy on rubella immunization is similar to that of the UK[35].

Between 15 and 19 years of age, booster doses of tetanus toxoid and poliomyelitis vaccine are recommended and offered to all senior pupils at school in the UK.

references

1. Tanner, J. M. (1962). *Growth at Adolescence.* (Oxford: Blackwell Scientific Publications)
2. Marshall, W. A. and Tanner, J. M. (1969). Variations in the pattern of pubertal changes in girls. *Arch. Dis. Child.*, **44**, 291
3. Marshall, W. A. and Tanner, J. M. (1970). Variations in the pattern of pubertal changes in boys. *Arch. Dis. Child.*, **45**, 13
4. Schofield, M. (1968). *The Sexual Behaviour of Young People.* (London: Penguin Books)
5. Wynne Davies, R. (1968). Familial idiopathic scoliosis. A family survey. *J. Bone Jt. Surg.*, **50B**, 24
6. Nachemson, A. (1968). A long term follow-up study of non-treated scoliosis. *Acta Orthopaed. Scand.*, **39**, 466
7. Nilsonne, U. and Lundgren, K. D. (1968). Long term prognosis in idiopathic scoliosis. *Acta Orthopaed. Scand.*, **39**, 456
8. Field, J. H. (1976). *Epidemiology of Head Injuries in England and Wales.* (London: HMSO)
9. Potter, J. M. (1973). Hospital admissions after head injury. *Lancet*, **1**, 1381
10. Symonds, C. (1962). Concussion and its sequelae. *Lancet*, **1**, 1
11. Erikson, E. H. M. (1964). *Insight and Responsibility.* (New York: Norton)
12. Rutter, M., Graham, P., Chadwick, O. F. D. and Yule, W. (1976). Adolescent turmoil: fact or fiction. *J. Child Psychol. Psychiatry*, **17**, 35
13. Donovan, E. and Adelson, J. (1966). *The Adolescent Experience.* (New York: John Wiley)
14. Wood, M. (1973). *Children: the Development of Personality and Behaviour.* (London: Harrap)
15. Mead, M. (1958). Adolescence in primitive and modern society. In Macoby, E. E., Newcombe, T. M. and Hartley E. L. (eds.) *Readings in Social Psychology.* (New York: Henry Holt)
16. Wolkind, S. N. and Coleman, J. C. (1976). The psychiatry of ado-

lescence. *Br. J. Hosp. Med.*, **16**, 575
17. Rutter, M., Tizard, J. and Whitmore, K. (1970). *Education, Health and Behaviour.* (London: Longman)
18. Britchnell, J. (1970). The relation between attempted suicide, depression and parental death. *Br. J. Psychiatry*, **116**, 307
19. Freour, P. *et al.* (1977). A survey of 2000 adolescents to determine the impact of the anti-smoking campaign in France. *Rev. Int. Educ. Sante*, **20**, 182
20. Exbroyat, J. (1977). Two investigations of childhood and alcoholism: a contribution to health education. *Rev. Hyg. Scol. Univ.*, **30**, 153
21. Banks, M. H. *et al.* (1978). Long term study of smoking by secondary schoolchildren. *Arch. Dis. Child.*, **53**, 12
22. Wolkind, S. N., Kruk, S. and Chaves, L. (1976). Childhood separation experiences and psychosocial status in primiparous women: preliminary findings. *Br. J. Psychiatry*, **128**, 391
23. OPCS (1978). *Abortion Statistics 1974, Schoolgirl Pregnancies: a first report.* British Pregnancy Advisory Service, Solihull, England
24. Hellman, L. (1973). *Pentimento.* (New York: Little)
25. *Report of the Committee on the Working of the Abortion Act* (1977). (London: HMSO)
26. Edwards, J. H. (1977). Heterozygote advantage. *Arch. Dis. Child.*, **52**, 343
27. Ratner, G. A. (1977). The coming of the second genetic code: eugenic abortion in the United Kingdom. In Raine, D. N. (ed). *Medico-Social Management of Inherited Metabolic Disease* (Lancaster: MTP Press)
28. Transport and Road Research Laboratory (1975). *Motorcycle Accidents and Injuries.* (London: HMSO)
29. Road Traffic Act 1972, (London: HMSO)
30. Maxcy-Rosenau (1973). In Sartwell, P. E. (ed.) *Preventive Medicine and Public Health.* (New York: Appleton-Century-Crofts)
31. Hart, P. D. A., and Sutherland, I. (1977). BCG and Vole bacillus vaccines in the prevention of tuberculosis in adolescence and early adult life: final report to the Medical Research Council. *Br. Med. J.*, **2**, 293
32. Morley, D. (1973). *Paediatric Priorities in the Developing World.* (London: Butterworth)
33. Comstock, G. W., Livesay, V. T. and Woolpert, S. F. (1974). Evaluation of BCG vaccination among Puerto Rican children. *Am. J. Pub. Health*, **64**, 283
34. Springett, V. H. (1976). Do we need BCG vaccination? *Postgrad. Med. J.*, **52**, 584
35. Report on a Working Group with the participation of the International Children's Centre (1977). *Immunisation Programmes for Children.* (Copenhagen: World Health Organisation)

chapter eight

child care services

child guidance service

In 1955, following the report of the Underwood Committee[1], Local Education Authorities (LEA's) were advised to establish a comprehensive child guidance service involving the school psychological service, the school health service and the child psychiatric service. The school psychological service is based in the LEA's child guidance clinic. In some authorities, the services of the school psychological service are extended to the pre-school child especially for those children with recognizable handicap or serious emotional disorder.

The child guidance clinics operate an 'open door' system and will accept referral of cases from any professional in the education, health or social services as well as accepting parents or older children themselves. Some Area Health Authorities have a specialist service for the pre-school child in addition to the hospital child psychiatric service, which extends psychiatric, psychological and social work support to parents whose very young children have emotional or behavioural problems, whether or not these are associated with physical or sensory handicap.

The child guidance team consists of a child psychiatrist, psychologist and psychiatric social worker. In the school psychological service the psychologist will be an educational psychologist: in the hospital department, the psychologist will be a clinical psychologist. The educational psychologist, whose background experience is in teaching and education, will not have the therapeutic skills of the clinical psychologist; likewise the clinical psychologist, who has no access to or experience with schools, is not able to manage fully the problems of children with educational difficulties[2].

In the care of the adolescent, there has been a gradual trend, reinforced by the report of the Committee on the Child Health Services[3], towards the integration of child and adolescent psychiatric services, although the special adolescent psychiatric units have brought about an improvement in the understanding and treatment of adolescent psychiatric disorder. There is a need for the treatment of young adolescents to be integrated into the psychiatric services provided for children, as disorder in young adolescents is usually an extension of childhood disturbance, whilst the older adolescent, in the 16 to 19 age group, is seen to require the same services as those provided for adults.

Children with physical handicap have an increased incidence of psychiatric disorder[4] which is higher in those children with severe sensory handicap when physical handicap is due to a neurological lesion such as cerebral palsy and epilepsy. The provision of child psychiatry for children who are profoundly deaf is scarce, there being only two specialist units in the United Kingdom. The child who is mentally handicapped is 3 to 4 times more likely to suffer psychiatric disorder[4], and in the severely mentally handicapped child, psychoses and serious mental illness are more common than in the general child population. The severely mentally handicapped schoolchild in need of psychiatric help will receive treatment from a psychiatrist in mental subnormality, not a child psychiatrist.

psychological tests

Most psychologists will use a variety of tests with individual children and issue a report giving a comprehensive view of the child's potential rather than an intelligence quotient which may not reflect the child's ability. When working with a psychologist, one should have an understanding of the tests they use, and, to obtain this, it is worthwhile sitting in on a test session with the psychologist.

The most common tests in use are the Wechsler Intelligence Scale for Children[5] (WISC), which has an age range of 5 to 15 years, and the Wechsler Pre-School and Primary Scale of Intelligence[6] (WPPSI) which has an age range of 4 to 6½ years. Both these scales give a separate result for verbal and performance intelligence and the report will show, e.g.

Verbal Scale (VS) : IQ 96
Performance Scale (PS) : IQ 103
Full Scale (FS) : IQ 99

The verbal and the performance scales may be administered separately, as in the case of those children who have a physical handicap, have speech and language problems or do not speak the English language.

Other tests in use include the Stanford–Binet Intelligence Scale[7], the age range of which is 2 years to adulthood. A major criticism of this test is that it has a verbal bias and it is becoming less popular with psychologists as it is used by many people who are not trained psychologists. The result of the test gives the intelligence quotient.

The Goodenough–Harris Drawing Test[8] has an age range of 3 to 15 years. The child is asked to make a picture of a man and the scoring is based on a 73 point scale, taking into account details of body, clothing and body proportions. This is a useful screening test but is not definitive.

Raven's Matrices[9] has an age range from 5½ years to adulthood. The test consists of a series of designs or matrices, each with a missing part, and the child has to choose which of a set of alternatives should be used to complete the design. The designs progress in complexity.

For babies and very young children, the tests most commonly in use are Gesell's test[10] of linguistic, adaptive and social behaviour, and the Ruth Griffiths test[11,12] covering the locomotor, personal–social, hearing–speech, eye–hand and performance scales for the 0- to 2-year-olds and including an additional scale for practical reasoning in the tests for the 2- to 8-year-old child. Both these scales give a development quotient (DQ) not an intelligence quotient (IQ). The Griffiths test is the one most commonly used by senior clinical doctors in the school and pre-school service and by paediatricians interested in developmental paediatrics. The material is attractive to babies and young children and can be used as part of a neurological examination in assessing co-ordination and fine movement and screening for sensory handicap. The test contains a picture vocabulary test which is simple to administer.

Both the Gesell and the Griffiths test may give a DQ within the normal range for a baby with mental handicap when that baby has had a good, stimulating environment. In such a case, credit should be given to the parents for the quality of their care, but the result of the test must be given with due caution about the probable outcome of later testing, when the level of more complex speech and language development in the second and third years comes under scrutiny. It is tragic for parents to be led to believe that their children are more capable than can be predicted at the time of testing, and in the young infant prediction is very limited. False impressions gained by parents lead to serious problems with later counselling especially when decisions are made about the type of school best suited to the child's needs.

The Peabody Picture Vocabulary Test[13], often referred to as the Peabody, is sometimes used as a test of intelligence although it was designed as a measure of hearing vocabulary and is in essence a language test.

Speech therapists also use a wide range of tests on children's speech and language. Again it is worthwhile asking the speech therapist if you may sit with the therapist when he/she is testing a patient. The most commonly used tests are the Reynell Development Language Scale[14] (referred to as the Reynell) and the Illinois Test of Psycholinguistic Abilities (ITPA)[15]. For testing language function, the speech therapist may use the Edinburgh Articulation Test or the Reed Test of Auditory Discrimination[16]. A recent study[17], comparing the Peabody and the auditory subtest of the ITPA as measures of auditory discrimination in 48 normal and 48 mentally retarded children, found that the Peabody was not an adequate measure of hearing vocabulary for mentally retarded children.

the school health service

Following the Elementary Education Act of 1870[18] and the introduction of compulsory education in 1880[19], many children were found to be unable to attend school or to benefit from their education due to poverty, ill-health or handicap, which led to the introduction of the school health service. In 1906, Local Education Authorities (LEA's) were given the power to provide free school meals[20], and, in 1907, medical examination of all children at school became compulsory[21]. These provisions were re-enacted in the 1944 Education Act[22] and the LEA's employed doctors, nurses, speech therapists and physiotherapists to fulfil their responsibilities under that Act which required the Education Authority to provide medical examination and treatment of all children attending school.

Following the re-organization of the National Health Service in 1974, the school health service and the public health service were transferred to the National Health Service (NHS) and the management of these services was delegated to the Area Health Authorities (AHA's). The public health service had been responsible for the developmental screening of the pre-school child, immunization, health visiting services and, with the school health service, the surveillance of children in the care of the local authority. Under the 1974 Act of Re-organisation[23], each AHA has a duty to provide medical and nursing services for nursing mothers and young children and a medical and dental service for pupils in schools. The Area Specialist for Child Health has a particular responsibility to the Local Education Authority for the medical and paramedical services provided for pupils in school, as the Area Nurse (Child Health) has for the nursing services and the Area Dental Officer has for dental services.

The aim of the school health service is to allow each child to take advantage of the education offered by ensuring that acute and chronic illness is treated and any physical, psychological or sensory handicap is alleviated as far as possible and is understood by the parents, child and teacher. School doctors work closely with teachers and psychologists in investigating and relieving the educational disadvantages associated with disability or handicap. School doctors will advise parents whose children have outstanding gifts and abilities and, with psychologists and teachers, recommend to the Education Authority any special provision, whether ordinary, special school or private education, that may be necessary.

Among the statutory responsibilities incorporated in the 1944 Education Act and of special concern to the health service, is the duty laid upon each LEA to ascertain all handicapped children by the age of 2 years who may be in need of special education. Doctors who examine children 'suffering from a disability of mind' must have special qualifications and experience[24]. These doctors will either have successfully completed a postgraduate course in child development and handicap or will be child psychiatrists working in a child guidance clinic.

Following the 1970 Education Act[25], severely mentally handicapped children were brought into the special education service with compulsory school attendance. Previously, this group of children had been cared for by the public health departments and attended occupation or training centres. Due to lack of facilities for assessment and funds for buildings and staff, many of these children, prior to 1971, were denied the advantages of attending the centres and their parents were denied a respite from care. The transfer of responsibility for this group of children to the LEA has undoubtedly been beneficial for the children. Schools were made available with trained teaching staff. Improved assessment – medical, educational and psychological – is provided for the children, with improved guidance and follow-up for the family. Senior centres for school leavers and adults are run by the Social Services Department and social workers are responsible for continuing to give support and help to the family.

Parents have the right to ask the Education Authority for an examination of their child from the age of two years if they think he may be in need of special education. Equally, parents have the right to appeal, by writing to the Secretary of State for Education and Science, if they disagree with the decision of the LEA that their child is in need of special education and should attend a special school[22].

The 1944 Education Act[23] designated children in need of special education on a medical model and did not include the schools in use in penal establishments and so excluded from their specialist care children in trouble with the law. Children with a physical or mental handicap who may need special education are examined by a senior medical officer of the School Health Service and assessed by a psychologist from the Education Service who will jointly, in collaboration with the class teacher, recommend to the LEA an appropriate school for the child. Children with sensory handicaps must be seen by the appropriate specialist; the paediatrician or senior school medical officer should also examine these children as single handicaps are uncommon and associated handicaps may be a more serious problem for the child, the family and the school.

Children who are visually handicapped must have a recommendation completed by their consultant ophthalmologist. The form in use was designed for adults who are blind or partially sighted and is unsuitable for children as it may be extremely difficult to decide if very young children are educationally blind, i.e. that they cannot be taught by sighted methods, or that they are partially sighted. Assessment of visually handicapped children needs to be improved from the point of view of the whole child not just their visual handicap.

The observations of the trained teacher of the visually handicapped is often of clinical importance to the consultant's review. Special schools for visually handicapped children are usually separate, depending on whether the children are blind or partially sighted, although more schools for the partially sighted have teachers of Braille on their staff and are able to accept children who are educationally blind.

Children with a hearing handicap (either profoundly deaf or partially hearing) must have a recommendation completed by the consultant otologist who will also prescribe the child's hearing aid. The observations of the teacher of the deaf and their co-operation in the management of the prescribed aid as well as advice and counselling for the parents is the usual pattern in good centres of paediatric otology, unlike the present position of the child with a visual handicap. The profoundly deaf child, who may or may not be able to learn by verbal methods, will usually attend either a day or residential special school. The units for the partially hearing child, who can be taught by verbal methods, are usually attached to ordinary schools.

With both vision- and hearing-handicapped children, the lines of demarcation between blindness and partial sight and between profound deafness and partial hearing, and the educational problems that may be involved, are very difficult to judge even for the most experienced professional in medicine or education. A more fluid and less doctrinaire approach to the type of education provided for these children, especially nursery education, and the form of teaching used, is becoming more common and, in the interests of the children, is to be applauded.

Children with speech and language disorders should be fully investigated by a consultant otologist before special education is decided upon. A simple hearing test is not adequate investigation. A report from the speech therapist is essential.

Children who are deemed maladjusted, whether due to a neurotic or behaviour disorder, will need confirmation of this diagnosis from a child psychiatrist, and the psychologist's and psychiatric social worker's reports should be made available to the receiving school. Since 1959, it has been the policy of the Education Department, now the Department of Education and Science, that children deemed maladjusted should live at home during their treatment and attend an ordinary school or a special school or class rather than be admitted to residential special schools[26]. If a boarding school is recommended in the interests of the child, for any reason, it is most helpful for the school to receive a social worker's assessment of the home background of the child.

The review of special education by the Warnock Committee[27] has suggested profound changes in attitudes to the needs of children for special education, seeking to embrace the wide range of children who have learning problems both in ordinary schools and special schools. Included in this concept are children committed to institutional care in community homes and so includes children who are in trouble with the law. Local Education Authorities have been asked to make available an educational and physical environment with the necessary aids, equipment and resources appropriate to the child's needs[27]. It has been estimated that one child in six needs this type of help at some time in their school life[2].

school medical examination

With improvement in the general health of the population, the necessity for every child in school to have a physical examination at intervals is in doubt. With competent screening of all pre-school children, necessary for the early treatment of physical and sensory handicap and psychiatric and psychological disorder, some form of selection for medical examination of the school child is sensible[28]. Apart from the follow-up of known handicap or disability and children who have serious intercurrent infection, illness or accident, selection for medical examination must be at two levels.

(1) At the request of the parents and teachers of pupils in a specific age group, e.g. 7+ years and 14+ years. Selection of specific age groups is necessary. Although parents, teachers and other professionals may initiate a request for a medical examination at any time, some parents and inex-

perienced teachers may be too shy to ask for advice or learn to live with the child's problem to the detriment of the child. In large schools, knowledge of individual children may be slight. Those children with the most serious psychological problems are adept at registering as attending school and then truanting. A formal request to teachers reminding them of individual children, their behaviour and work record is often helpful.

(2) At the request of the school nurse. The school nurse sees each child at regular intervals at school for vision testing and for surveys of each child's general health and development. The nurse will make home visits when there is a problem relating to the child's health in school or failed appointments for specialist clinics. The nurse will be known to those parents in need of additional support and will be better known and more accessible to the individual class teacher than the school doctor, as the latter will be covering a much wider range of work.

Speech therapists and physiotherapists are an integral part of the school health service and children attending for therapy will be reviewed by the school doctor, preferably with the therapist.

On visiting a school, the doctor or nurse will always see the head teacher. Parents are always invited to attend when their children are seen by the school doctor but not at the more frequent health screening of the school nurse. There are occasions when parents are not able to attend the medical examination and other times when it is necessary to examine children without their parents, as in a case of non-accidental injury. When parents are not able to attend, it is courteous to write and tell the parents that the examination has taken place and what the outcome is. Children's love, affection and loyalty for their parents should never be undermined, nor their affection for their teacher and loyalty to their school, although disturbance of these emotions in the child may be the cause of behaviour disorder. Senior pupils will prefer, and often insist upon, a private interview and medical examination and this should be made available to them.

General advice is made available in writing (see appendix 3) to all head teachers on the exclusion period and management of contacts when pupils have infectious diseases.

Another group of people with whom the doctor and nurse work are the officers of the Education Welfare Service. These officers follow up children who have been absent from school or who are recurrently absent. When absence is genuine and due to ill-health, the school doctor may be asked to review the child. It may be that the type of school or the distance travelled should be altered. Where the absence is feigned ill-health, it may be due to true school phobia or truancy. In either case, where psychological disorder is present, the child will be referred to the Child Guidance Clinic or to the Hospital Child Psychiatric Clinic. If truancy persists recourse may be had to legal powers[22] vested in the Education Authority to ensure school attendance.

references

1. DHSS (1955). *Report of the Committee on Maladjusted Children,* (London: HMSO)
2. Rutter, M., Tizard, J. and Whitmore, K. (eds.) (1970). *Education, Health and Behaviour.* (London: Longman)
3. Report of the Committee on the Child Health Services (1976). *Fit for the Future* (London: HMSO)
4. Rutter, M. (1975). *Helping Troubled Children.* (London: Penguin Books)
5. Wechsler, D. (1949). *Wechsler Intelligence Scale for Children, Manual.* (New York: The Psychological Corporation)
6. Wechsler, D. (1967). *Wechsler Pre-school and Primary Scale of Intelligence, Manual* (New York: The Psychological Corporation)
7. Terman, L. M. and Merrill, M. A. (1961) *Stanford–Binet Intelligence Scale: Manual for the Third Revision.* (London: Harrap)
8. Harris, D. B. (1963). *Children's Drawings as Measures of Intellectual Maturity.* (New York: Harcourt Brace and World)
9. Raven, J. C. (1965). *Guide to Using the Coloured Progresssive Matrices.* (London: Lewis)
10. Gesell, A. (1925). *The Mental Growth of the Pre-School Child.* (New York: Macmillan)
11. Griffiths, R. (1954). *The Abilities of Babies.* (London: University of London Press)
12. Griffiths, R. (1970). *The Abilities of Young Children.* (London: Child Development Research Centre)

13. Dunn, L. M. (1959). *Peabody Picture Vocabulary Test.* (Circle Pines, Minnesota: American Guidance Service)
14. Reynell, J. K. (1969). *Test Manual. Reynell Development Language Scales.* (London: National Foundation for Educational Research)
15. McCarthy, J. J. and Kirk, S. A. (1961). *Illinois Test of Psycholinguistic Abilities.* (Urbana, Illinois: University of Illinois)
16. Reed, M. (1960). *Reed Test of Auditory Discrimination.* (London: Royal National Institute for the Deaf)
17. Williams, A. M., Marks, C. J. and Bialer, I. (1977). Validity of the Peabody picture vocabulary test as a measure of hearing vocabulary in mentally retarded and normal children. *J. Speech Hear.*, **20**, 205
18. Elementary Education Act, 1870 (London: HMSO)
19. Elementary Education Act, 1880. (London: HMSO)
20. Education (Provision of Meals) Act, 1906. (London: HMSO)
21. Education (Administrative Provisions) Act, 1907. (London: HMSO)
22. Education Act, 1944. (London: HMSO)
23. National Health Service Re-organisation Act, 1973. (London: HMSO)
24. National Health Service (Medical Examinations – Educationally Subnormal Children) Regulations, 1974. (London: HMSO)
25. Education (Handicapped Children) Act, 1970. (London: HMSO)
26. Ministry of Education, Circular 348. (1959). *Special Educational Treatment for Maladjusted Children.* (London: HMSO)
27. Report of the Committee of Enquiry into the Education of Handicapped Children and Young People. (1978). *Special Educational Needs.* (London: HMSO)
28. Ashley-Miller, M. (1965). Selective school medical inspection. *Med. Officer*, **113**, 119

appendix one

hearing tests

The aim of all hearing tests is to assess whether the child can discriminate the relative loudness of the vowel sounds found in the low frequencies and the soft or unvoiced consonants found in the high frequencies. This discrimination is necessary for the development of normal speech.

The principles involved in testing babies are the use of the high tone *ss* sound, the low tone *oo* sound, a high frequency rattle, a low frequency rattle or a voiced phrase that appeals to the infant. All the sounds are delivered at 30–35 dB and the level of ambient noise recorded by a sound meter. Two people are necessary when carrying out the test on infants and young children. While the baby sits on the mother's lap, one person acts to distract the infant and to observe the infant's response to the delivery of sounds by the tester who is behind and to the side of the infant.

Babies who fail this test may have a congenital or sensorineural deafness (see figure 7), and are referred to a special clinic where the baby can be retested in a sound attenuated room using sounds similar to those used previously and free field audiometry. Staff involved in testing the hearing of infants by these methods should have normal hearing so that their voiced sounds are not too loud. Regular screening of the hearing of personnel with pure tone audiometry should be undertaken.

In the older, more co-operative child, hearing tests can be carried out by a wide variety of methods. Experience and knowledge of children's reactions is important in assessing results. Some tests can be used in the consulting room, others need skilled personnel and special facilities.

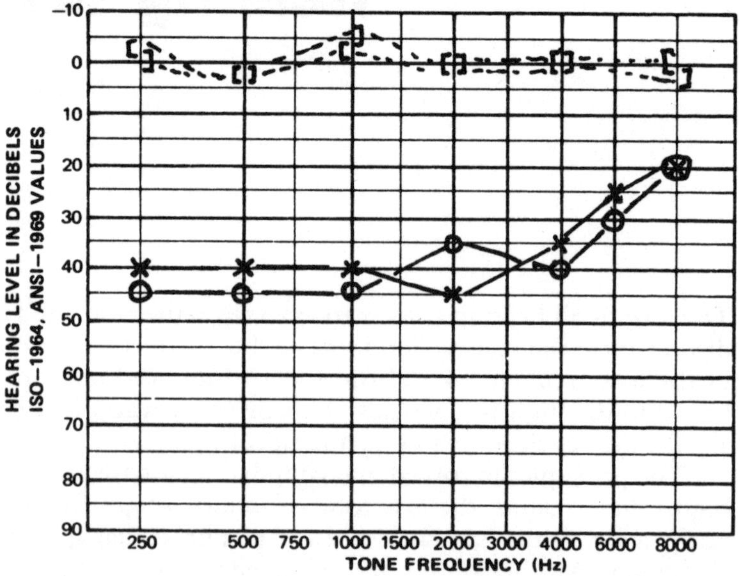

figure 6
audiograms showing conductive loss; right ear: air conduction o—o, bone conduction [—[; left ear: air conduction ×—×, bone conduction]—]

Weber test

The vibrating tuning fork is placed on the vertex or the forehead and the patient asked which ear hears more clearly. In conductive deafness (see figure 6), the sound is lateralized to the worse ear. In sensori-neural deafness (see figure 7), the sound is lateralized to the better ear. The test is indicated in unilateral or unequal deafness.

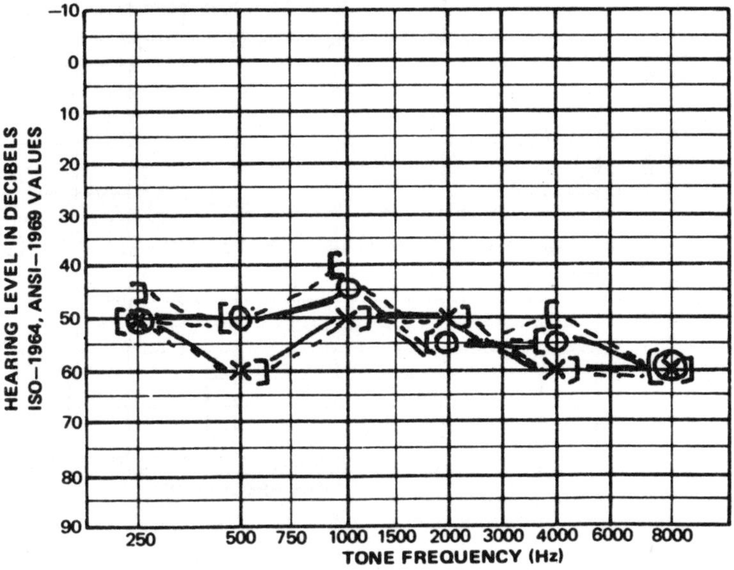

figure 7
audiogram showing sensori-neural loss; key as figure 6

Rinné test

The vibrating tuning fork is held near but not touching the ear and the patient indicates when the sound is no longer heard. This tests air conduction (AC) (see figure 6). With children, it is simpler to ask them which is the louder or the point to where the sound was louder.

In sensori-neural deafness and in the normal ear, AC is better than BC. This is a positive Rinné. In conductive deafness, BC is better than AC (see figure 6). This is a negative

Rinné. In some cases of unilateral sensori-neural loss, the sound travels through the skull to the good cochlea, giving a false negative Rinné. To prevent such misleading results the good ear should be masked by a Barany noise box (see figure 8).

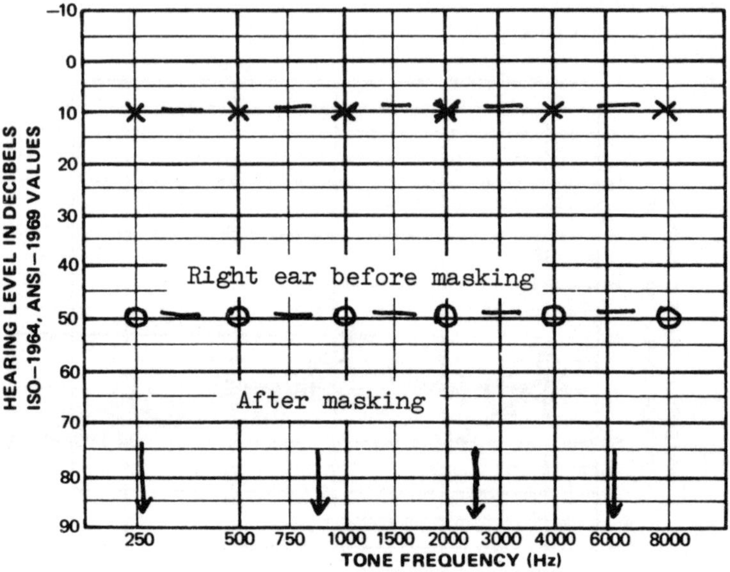

figure 8
audiogram showing unilateral hearing loss, demonstrating the result of masking with a Barany noise box; key as figure 6

the Schwarbach test of absolute bone conduction (ABC)

This test is used to diagnose unilateral sensori-neural deafness, Rinné positive. The stem of the vibrating tuning fork is placed on the patient's mastoid process and the bone conduction time compared with the examiner's, always presuming that the otologist's hearing is normal. Ambient noise is excluded by pressing the tragus into the meatus. The test may be carried out with high and low tone forks to assess the level of the loss (see figures 9 and 10).

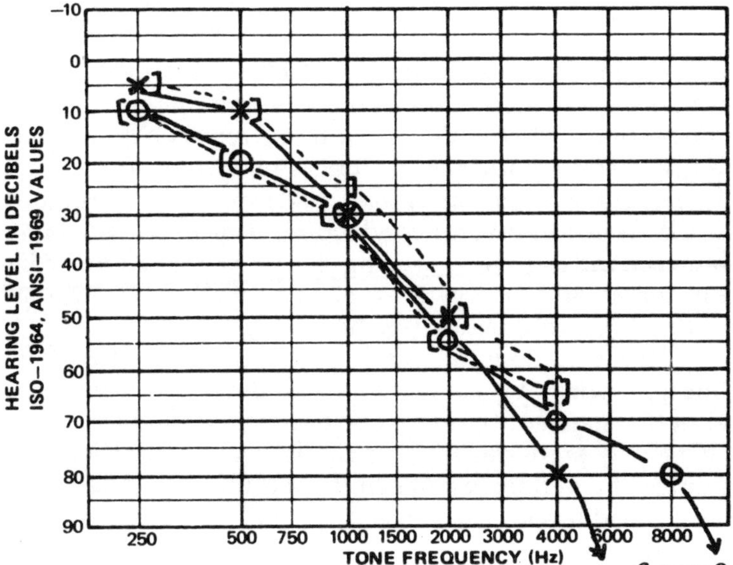

figure 9
audiogram showing high tone loss – 'ski-type'; key as figure 6

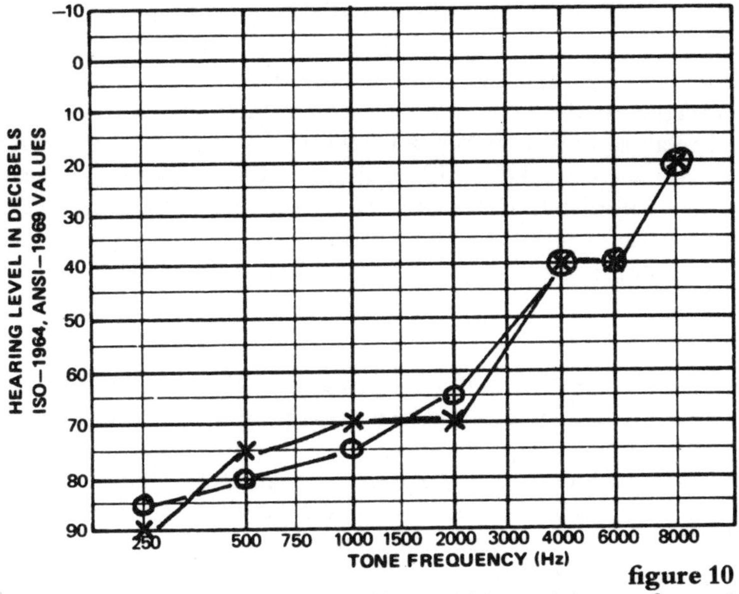

figure 10
audiogram showing low tone loss – 'ski-type'; key as figure 6

pure tone audiometry

The range of normal hearing is 125 Hz to 6000–8000 Hz for air conduction, which is the conductive mechanism, and bone conduction, which is the cochlear and retrocochlear function. When testing with a pure tone audiometer, the effects of ambient or background noise may lower the threshhold by 20 dB. When testing air conduction, if there is a gap of 40 dB between the two ears, masking should be applied to the better ear and should always be applied to the opposite ear when testing bone conduction (see figure 11).

On the audiogram, the presence of a space between the lines showing air conduction and bone conduction is the air–bone gap (see figure 6) and indicates a conductive loss. If the gap is predominantly in the lower tones, there may be fluid in the middle ear. When there is no gap between air and bone conduction, then sensori-neural, or perceptive, loss is present.

Pure tone audiometry is used to sweep test large numbers of children in school at 5, 9 and 14 years of age. Any hearing loss found is reviewed by the school doctor and audiometrician 4 to 6 weeks later, with a report to the family doctor. If the hearing loss is confirmed on retest, the child will be referred to the special clinic where further testing, by pure tone audiometry or other methods, in soundproofed booths or rooms is available. The patient will be seen by the consultant otologist if necessary. If serious or permanent hearing impairment is found, the child will be followed up in school by the audiometrician and the teacher of the deaf.

impedance testing

Impedance testing is used when a normal drum is found in association with a conductive loss on pure tone audiometry (see figure 11). The nerve supply to the stapedius must be intact as the impedance test measures the stapedius reflex and gives imformation on recruitment and non-organic deafness. A probe containing three fine tubes is inserted into the external meatus so that an airtight seal is obtained. The tubes convey pure tone noise from the audiometer to the eardrum; the

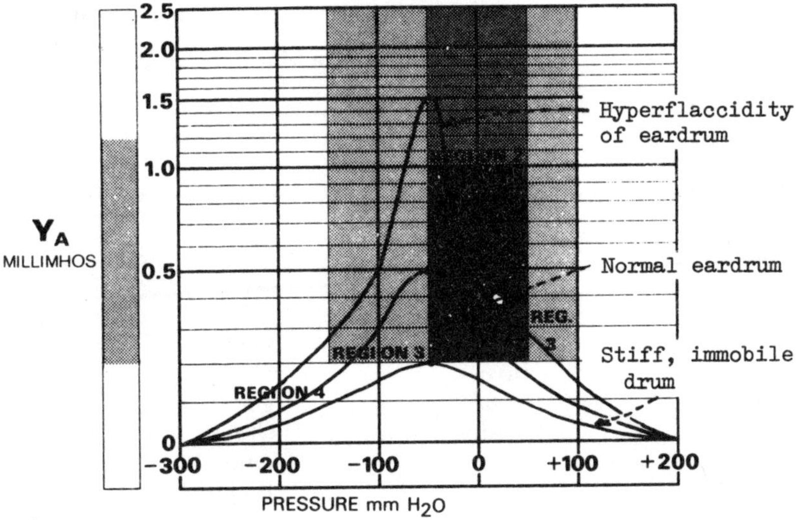

figure 11
impedance test results

reflected sound from the drum to the impedance meter and the air from a pump can increase and decrease the pressure in the external auditory meatus, thus testing the seal and also calibrating the plotter. The results of impedance testing show the elasticity or compliance of the drum and the middle ear mechanism by the shape of the curve plotted. A steep curve at zero indicates increased elasticity or decreased impedance and occurs in ossicular discontinuity. A shift of the curve to the left of zero shows decreased elasticity or increased impedance, as more energy is bounced back to the impedance meter. This occurs in glue ear. A further shift to the left indicates a blockage of the Eustachian tube. A low curve indicates otosclerosis.

The level of the stapedial reflex is plotted at various frequencies on an audiometry graph with the pure tone threshold. The closer together the two lines become, the more recruitment is taking place and cochlear sensori-neural deafness is confirmed. If the lines are very close together, this will indicate to the hearing aid technician that a hearing aid with the necessary volume to correct the loss may cause

table 8

the Manchester Word Test

No. 1	*ear*	*dB*	*%*	*No. 2*	*ear*	*dB*	*%*	*No. 3*	*ear*	*dB*	*%*
ship				fish				thud			
rug				duck				witch			
fan				gap				wrap			
cheek				cheese				jail			
haze				rail				keys			
dice				hive				vice			
both				bone				get			
well				wedge				shown			
lot				moss				hoof			
move				tooth				bomb			

No. 4	*ear*	*dB*	*%*	*No. 5*	*ear*	*dB*	*%*	*No. 6*	*ear*	*dB*	*%*
fun				fib				fill			
will				thatch				catch			
vat				sum				thumb			
shape				heel				heap			
wreath				wide				wise			
hide				rake				rave			
guess				goes				goat			
comb				shop				shone			
choose				vet				bed			
job				June				juice			

table 8 continued

No. 7	*ear*	*dB*	*%*	*No.* 8	*ear*	*dB*	*%*	*No.* 9	*ear*	*dB*	*%*
badge				bath				hush			
hutch				hum				gas			
pill				dip				thin			
thighs				five				fake			
save				ways				chime			
reap				reach				weave			
foam				joke				jet			
loose				noose				rob			
dot				got				dope			
shed				shell				lose			

No. 10	*ear*	*dB*	*%*	*No.* 11	*ear*	*dB*	*%*	*No.* 12	*ear*	*dB*	*%*
jug				man				have			
match				hip				whizz			
whip				thug				buff			
faith				ride				mice			
sign				siege				teeth			
bees				veil				gauge			
hell				chose				poach			
rod				shoot				rule			
vote				web				den			
shook				cough				cosh			

distortion and excessive discomfort to the wearer, and may be the reason the child takes off or switches off the hearing aid provided. If the stapedial reflex is not elicited, retrocochlear deafness is present as the reflex arc is broken.

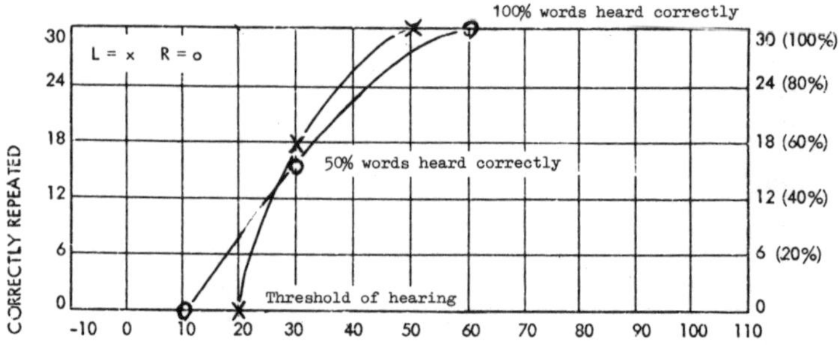

figure 12
speech audiogram

speech audiometry

This is used to test the patient's response to and ability to understand the spoken word compared with his appreciation of pure tones (see figure 12). It is particularly valuable in deciding on the patient's ability to use a hearing aid. The words used are phonetically balanced and the accuracy of response is plotted against intensity of sound. In conductive loss the graph follows the normal curve but at a higher intensity. A falling away curve indicates increasing inaccuracy, despite increasing intensity. This type of curve is characteristic of recruitment, so that speech brought to an audible level is merely made more difficult to decipher.

screening test for speech heard

The Manchester Junior Word Test (table 8) enables the doctor to screen a child's ability to hear words accurately. Each list contains 30 speech sounds. A 5-year-old should be able to repeat 92% of the sounds correctly and a 9-year-old should be able to repeat 97% of the sounds correctly. To explain the test to the child, the child should face the tester and repeat one of the lists of words after him. The tester must speak slowly, clearly and distinctly allowing the child to see his face. The words must be spoken not read. This allows the child to gain confidence and of course no correction is made; if a word is repeated incorrectly by the child a similar speech sound is then given. This initial procedure also allows the examiner to become used to the child's manner of pronouncing words, so that the hearing test can be scored correctly and children with speech defects can be tested. The child should be told he will be asked to repeat other similar words but he will not be able to see the tester's face. The child is then seated on a chair 3 feet away from and side on to the examiner. The child is instructed to look straight ahead, *not* at his mother, and the other ear is occluded by the child or mother pressing the tragus into the meatus. A different list of words is repeated for each ear and each ear is tested separately.

auditory evoked response (AER)

These tests are available in a few highly specialized centres and are used to test the hearing of children and adults who are severely handicapped, in some cases to confirm the diagnosis where patients are unco-operative or unwilling to admit their hearing loss, and in cases of psychological hearing loss. The evoked potential produced by the sound is small and can be identified only after summation by a computer. Both the method of carrying out the test and the reading of the result requires a skilled technical department and a consultant in neurophysiology.

appendix two

developmental questionnaires

6 weeks

MOTOR

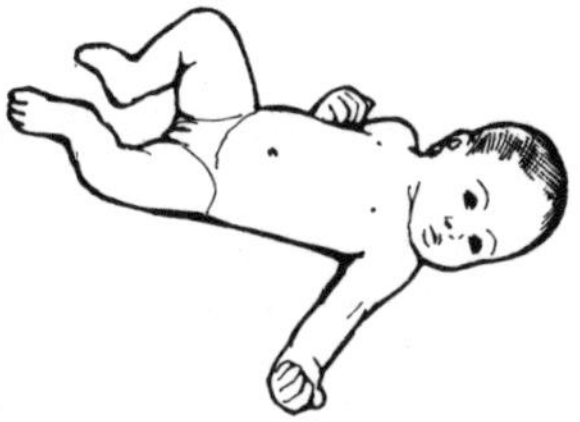

Supine
Head held to one side
yes/no

Supine
Limbs on that side
extended *yes/no*

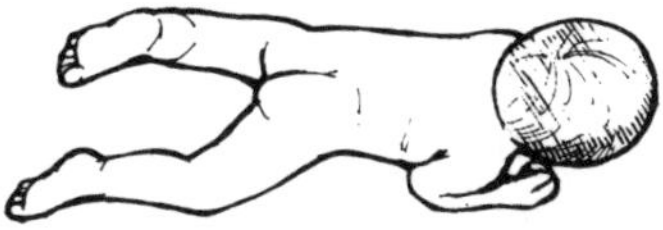

Prone
Pelvis flat, hips extended *yes/no*

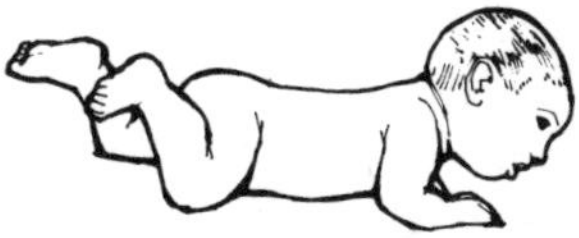

Prone
Lifts head momentarily
yes/no

Prone
Head lags when pulled to sit *yes/no*

VISION

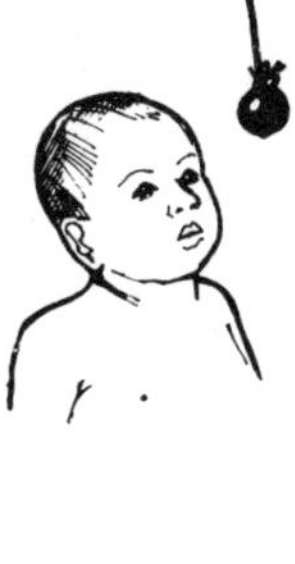

Follows dangling
8–10″ from side
to middle *yes/no*

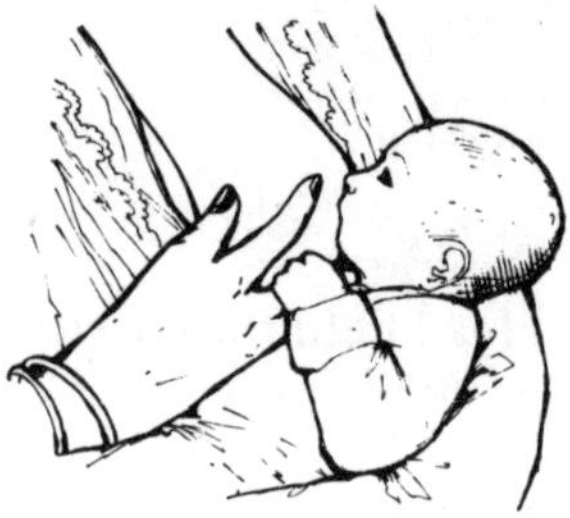

Watches mother's face during feeding *yes/no*

Social smile *yes/no*

HEARING AND SPEECH

Stills or turns eyes toward nearby speaker or bell *yes/no*

Startle to loud sound *yes/no*

Cries with discomfort *yes/no*

Coos responsively when pleased *yes/no*

SOCIAL AND FEEDING

Breast:
Bottle:
Excessive regurgitation or vomiting
Solids
Vitamins
Sleep
P.U.
Bowels
At home/D.N./child minder

PHYSICAL EXAMINATION

Normal *yes/no*

....
Medication ....
Parental care..
(incl. cleanliness)
Parents happy *yes/no*
Action...

SIGNATURE ....

6–8 months

MOTOR

Tone: normal/increased/diminished
Reflexes equal *yes/no*

Supine: lifts head, can bring legs vertical *yes/no*

Pulls to sit with
head held erect,
back straight
yes/no

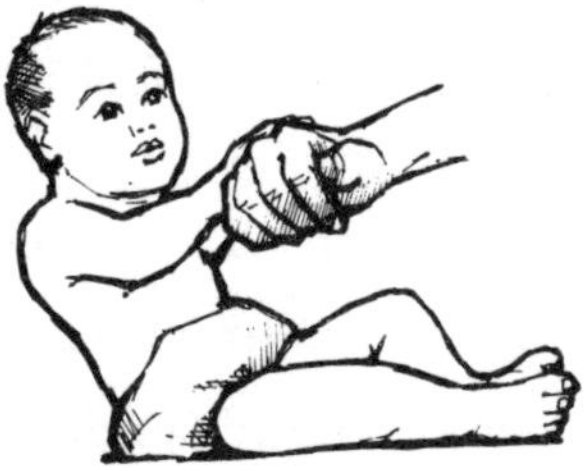

Prone
Lifts head and chest on extended arms
yes/no

Whole hand used
in palmar grasp
yes/no

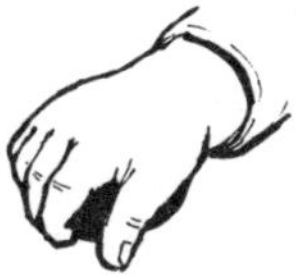

VISION

Full conjugate eye movements with head erect *yes/no*

Squint *yes/no*
Visually alert *yes/no*

Sees objects ½″
in diameter
(smartie) and
reaches for
yes/no

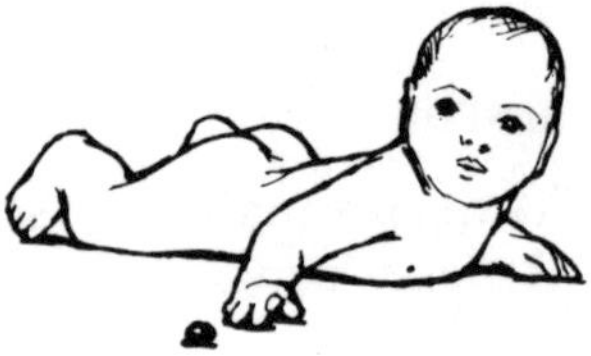

HEARING AND SPEECH

Localizes voice and sound-making objects (specify) at 1½ ft
yes/no

Vocalizes 1–2 syllables *yes/no*

Shouts for attention *yes/no*

Chuckles and laughs *yes/no*

SOCIAL AND FEEDING

Bottle/cup ....
Excessive regurgitation or vomiting
Solids
Vitamins
Sleep
P.U.
Bowels
At home/D.N./child minder

PHYSICAL EXAMINATION

Normal *yes/no*

....
Medication ....
Parental care..
(incl. cleanliness)
Parents happy *yes/no*
Action..

SIGNATURE ....

12 months

MOTOR

Sits well and
pivots *yes/no*

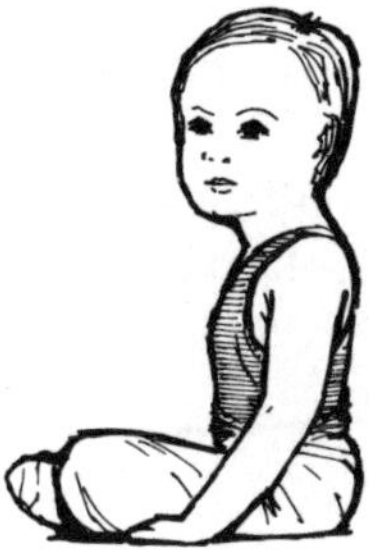

Crawls rapidly
or shuffles
yes/no

Can pull to stand and let self down
yes/no
Casts objects *yes/no*

Explores
yes/no

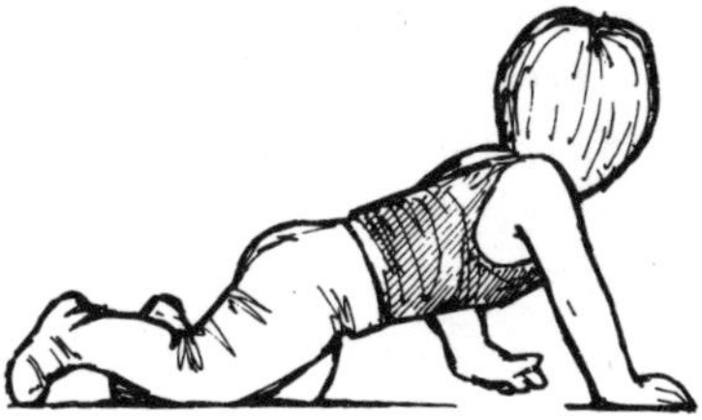

Finger thumb
apposition in
grasping cube
or pellet *yes/no*

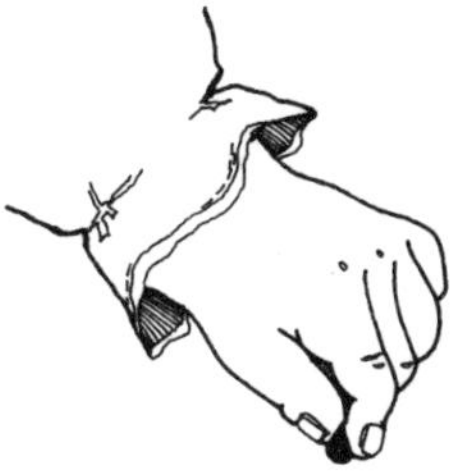

VISION

Squint *yes/no*

Follows dangling
ball in all
directions *yes/no*

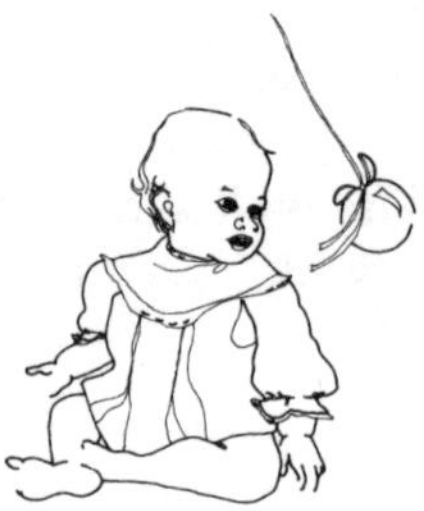

Picks up a pellet
(saccharine)
yes/no

Retrieves a toy
hidden before
his eyes under
a cup or cushion
yes/no

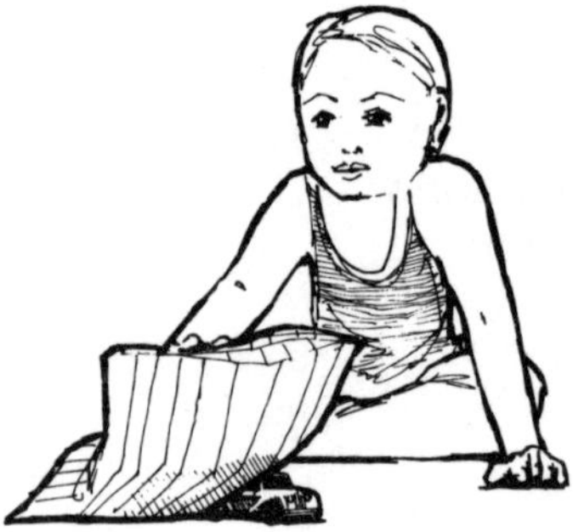

HEARING AND SPEECH

Knows and answers to own name *yes/no*

Babbles long repetitive strings of sounds *yes/no*

Obeys simple instruction 'give me', says 'bye-bye' *yes/no*

SOCIAL AND FEEDING

Bottle/cup..
Any regurgitation or vomiting
Meals: finger feeding
Vitamins
Sleep
P.U.
Bowels
At home/D.N./child minder

PHYSICAL EXAMINATION

Normal *yes/no*

....
Medication ....
Parental care...
(incl. cleanliness)
Parents happy *yes/no*
Action...

SIGNATURE ....

12/18 months to 2 years

MOTOR

Walks well *yes/no*
Runs *yes/no*

Can stoop, climbs
yes/no

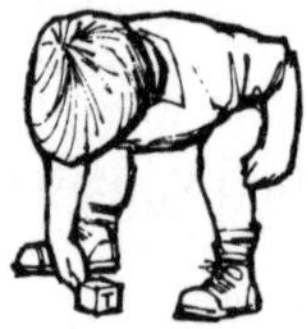

Can kick *yes/no*

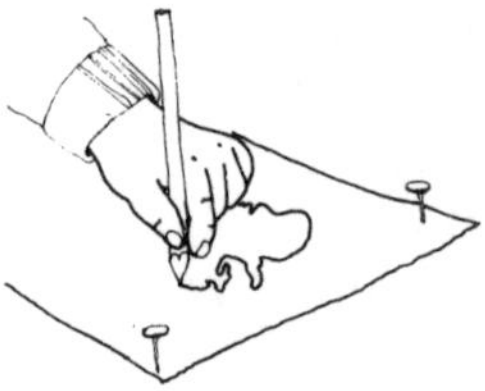

Scribbles with
preferred hand
left/right
yes/no

Describe – scribble, straight line, circle

VISION

Squint *yes/no*
Sees miniature toy at 10 ft *yes/no*

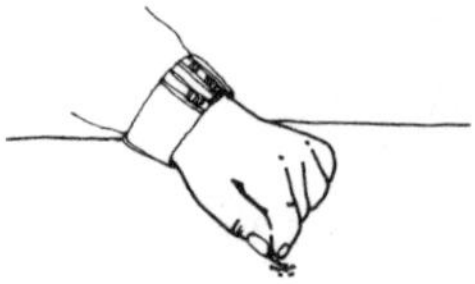

Picks up pellet
(hundreds and
thousands)
yes/no

Glasses *yes/no*

HEARING AND SPEECH

12+ clear words *yes/no*

Uses 2–3 word combinations *yes/no*

Gives first name *yes/no*

LANGUAGE AND SOCIAL

Talks continuously to self at play *yes/no*

Cleanliness asks *yes/no*

Dry during day *yes/no*

Likes to be near adults *yes/no*

Uses cup and spoon *yes/no*

At home/D.N./child minder

PHYSICAL EXAMINATION

Normal *yes/no*

....

Medication ....

Parental care..

(incl. cleanliness)

Parents happy *yes/no*

Action..

SIGNATURE ....

3 years

MOTOR

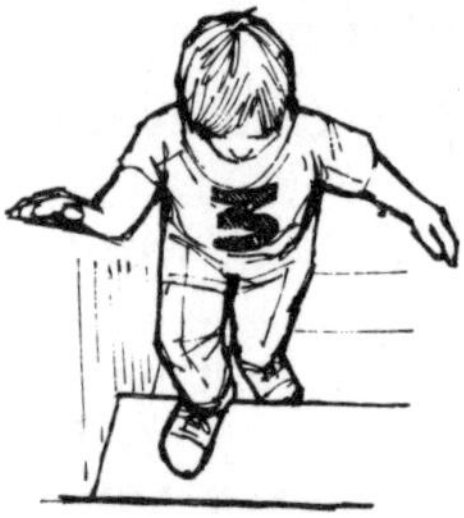

Walks upstairs
one foot on
each step
yes/no

Stands on one foot 6 seconds *yes/no*

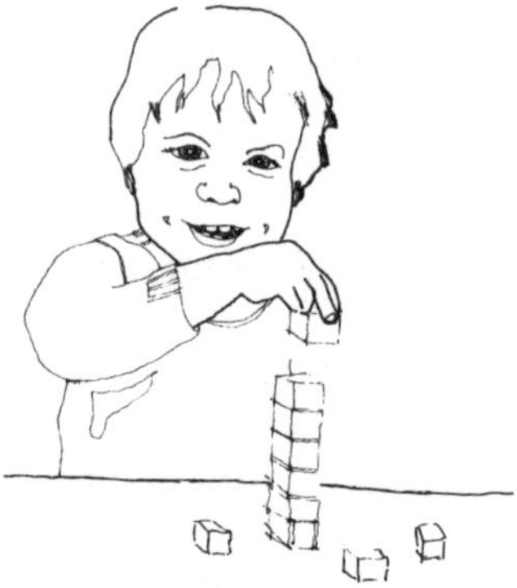

Brick tower (8)
yes/no

Tone

Reflexes

VISION

V/A Stycar* 5 letter card 10 ft
Squint *yes/no*
Near vision
(state test used)
(hundreds and thousands)
Glasses *yes/no*
Full conjugate movement with head erect *yes/no*

*Stycar Vision and Hearing Tests, NFER, Slough, England.

HEARING AND SPEECH

Picture vocabulary* test 6 high frequency words at 10 ft *yes/no*

Uses 6-syllable sentences *yes/no*

Can name familiar objects, toys and pictures *yes/no*

LANGUAGE AND SOCIAL

Defines by use (2) cup, spoon, chair, car, pencil *yes/no*

Gives first name on request *yes/no*

Uses spoon and fork *yes/no*

Dry/clean day and/or night *yes/no*

Parallel play *yes/no*

At home/D.N./N.S./child minder

PHYSICAL EXAMINATION

Normal *yes/no*

....

Medication ....

Parental care...

(incl. cleanliness)

Parents happy *yes/no*

Action...

SIGNATURE ....

4½ to 5 years

MOTOR

Can run fast *yes/no*

Can hop three
steps on one
foot *yes/no*

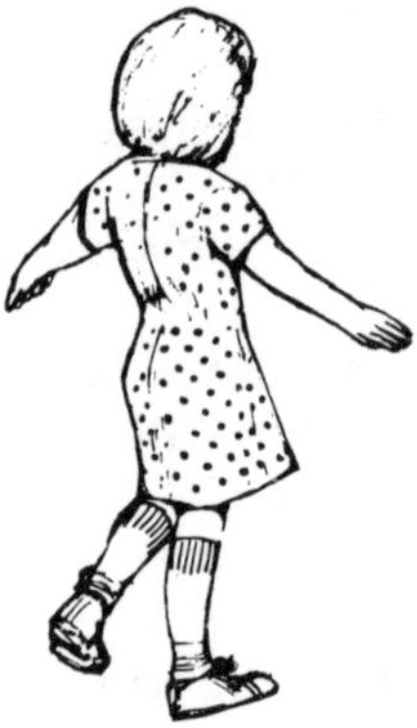

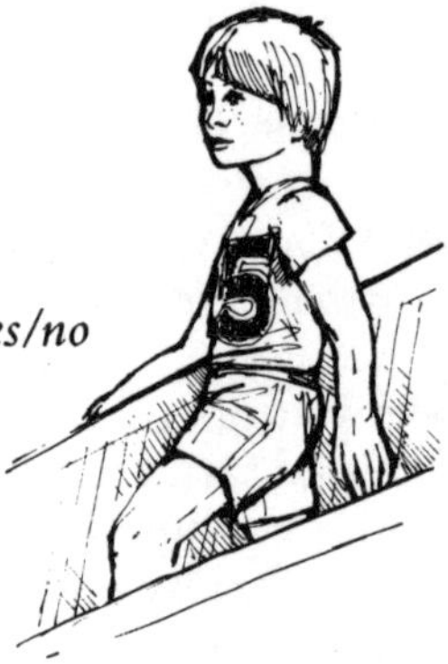

Can walk down
stairs one foot
at a time
yes/no

Can climb off and on bus unaided *yes/no*
Tone
Reflexes

VISION

V/A Stycar* 7–9 letter card at 20 ft
Squint *yes/no*
Near vision (state test used) (hundreds and thousands)
Colour vision *yes/no*
Glasses

*Stycar Vision and Hearing Tests, NFER, Slough, England

HEARING AND SPEECH

Articulation normal except for s/f/th sounds *yes/no*

Repeats list of words† each ear separately without lip reading *yes/no*
R *yes/no*
L *yes/no*

LANGUAGE AND SOCIAL

Knows name *yes/no*
age *yes/no*
address *yes/no*
Washes
Dresses
Preliminary counting to 4 *yes/no*
Plays well with other children *yes/no*
Knows sex *yes/no*
School: ordinary
special

PHYSICAL EXAMINATION

Normal *yes/no*
....
Medication ....
Parental care...
(incl. cleanliness)
Parents happy *yes/no*
Action..

SIGNATURE ....

†Manchester Word Test (table 8)

appendix three

data sheet on infectious diseases

Exclusion Periods of the Commoner Skin Infections

Disease	Minimal Period of Exclusion
Impetigo	Until skin is healed.
Pediculosis	Until treatment received.
Plantar Warts	Exclusion unnecessary.
Ringworm of Scalp	Until cured.
Ringworm of Body	No exclusion during treatment.
Ringworm of Feet (Athlete Foot)	Exclusion from bare foot activity unnecessary but treatment always advised.
Scabies	Exclusion unnecessary once adequate treatment is instituted.

(Revised November, 1977)

BIRMINGHAM AREA HEALTH AUTHORITY (TEACHING)

CHILD HEALTH SERVICE

INCUBATION AND EXCLUSION PERIODS OF THE COMMONER INFECTIOUS DISEASES

Disease	Usual Incubation Period (days)	Interval between onset and appearance of rash (days)	PERIOD OF EXCLUSION	
			Patients	Contacts, i.e. the other members of the family or household living together as a family, that is, in one dwelling.
Bacillary Dysentery	1 - 7	-	Until considered clinically fit by medical practitioner or at the discretion of the Specialist in Community Medicine /EH)	Siblings in primary and nursery school for 7 days. Older pupils should not be allowed to do domestic science(s) and handle food for 7 days.
Chickenpox	11 - 21	0 - 2	Usually until rash has healed and not less than 6 days from the onset of the rash.	None
Shingles	11 - 21	0 - 2	Until clinically fit.	None.
Diphtheria	2 - 5	-	Until considered by a medical practitioner to be fit and free from infection.	Return to school should not be permitted until bacteriological examination has proved negative.
Food Poisoning	2 - 48 hours		Please notify Specialist in Community Medicine (Environmental Health). (235 4642).	None.
German Measles	14 - 21	0 - 2	Until considered fit by medical practitioner but not less than 4 days from the onset of the rash.	None.
Glandular Fever	2 - 6 weeks		Until considered clinically fit by medical practitioner.	None.
Hepatitis A	15 - 50 (commonly 28)		7 days from onset of jaundice.	None. Older pupils should not be allowed to do domestic science and handle food for 7 days.
Measles	10 - 15	3 - 4	Until considered fit by medical practitioner but not before 7 days from the onset of the rash.	None unless the school child shows sign of upper respiratory infection, fever or cough.
Meningococcal Infection (Meningitis)	2 - 10	-	Until considered clinically fit by medical practitioner.	Excluded at the discretion of Specialists in Community Medicine (Environmental Health) &/or (Child Health).
Mumps	18 - 21	-	Until swelling has subsided. (7 days minimum).	None.
Poliomyelitis	3 - 21	-	Until considered clinically fit by medical practitioner.	Until considered fit by Specialists in Community Medicine (Child Health) and (Environmental Health).
Encephalitis	4 - 30	-		
Scarlet Fever (and Streptococcal sore throat)	2 - 5	1 - 2	Until appropriate treatment has been given and patient declared by medical practitioner fit to return.	None.
Whooping Cough	7 - 10		Until considered fit by medical practitioner but not less than 21 days from the onset of paroxysmal cough.	None.

index